STEPPING OUTSIDE THE BOX

A Journey from Invisible Pain to Invincible Living

Dr. Traci Patterson

Copyright © 2020 Traci A Patterson

Names and identifying details have been changed to protect
the privacy of individuals. This book is not intended as a
substitute for the medical advice of physicians. The reader
should regularly consult a physician in matters relating
to his/her health and particularly with respect to any
symptoms that may require diagnosis or medical attention.

ISBN-13: 978-0-578-71732-6

Cover design by: Traci Patterson
Printed in the United States of America

CONTENTS

Stepping Outside the Box

A Journey from Invisible Pain to Invincible Living

For everyone suffering with chronic pain, an invisible illness, Complex Regional Pain Syndrome (CRPS), their loved ones and care takers. May you be blessed with the courage and grace to find the strength and hope you deserve. Know there are answers and treatment options that can help.

FORWARD

Traci Patterson is a survivor. She writes with passion about her battles with and eventual victory over the severe pain of Complex Regional Pain Syndrome (CRPS). It all started with a seemingly minor ankle sprain and soon Traci was experiencing worsening pain and debility which traditional western treatments were unsuccessful in resolving. Investigating "all treatments known to the Internet" and trying many of them, Traci remained in severe pain. Her search for relief included many trips to Germany and Mexico which were temporarily helpful but ultimately did not get her into remission. Surgeries failed to give relief. Nerve blocks, physical therapy, spinal cord stimulators and an exceedingly long list of attempted treatments failed. Pain medications provided limited and incomplete relief. Finally, Traci experienced true success with a combination of treatments which included clinical hypnosis, neuroplasticity training, and working with the biology and physiology of the body.

Traci is now successfully treating other CRPS and chronic pain patients. Her protocol Hypnosis

Combined Therapy (HCT) is a comprehensive Intensive that is individualized to meet the specific needs and goals of each patient. Traci knows that results in healthcare cannot be guaranteed but her success in treating complicated and difficult pain conditions is impossible to ignore.

I recommend this book to those individuals living with CRPS and similar forms of chronic pain, their caregivers and all healthcare professionals who seek to better understand and help those with CRPS.

There IS hope.

Keith E. Davis, MD
Family Physician - Shoshone, Idaho
Idaho Physician of Year 2012
AAFP Physician of Year 2013
Top Doctor Award

PREFACE

Patients trust that their healthcare professionals will pause for a moment prior to entering the room to collect their thoughts and focus on what is important to the person they are about to see. People want to be heard and understood. Their pain is real, and they need solutions. They don't want to be told it's all in their head or not to worry. They want to trust their physician, clinician or healthcare provider will guide them in the right direction.

I trusted my doctors; especially the Podiatric surgeon that I had been so strongly referred to. Throughout the initial surgeries that he had completed, the months that turned into years of physical therapy, and many treatments I had to endure.

I relied on my surgeon. I believed him when he told me that I had Plantar Fasciitis; although I had been referred to him due to a severely sprained ankle that wasn't healing. We are taught to trust our doctors. They are supposed to be the experts and know what they are doing. The way my surgeon exuded himself; his strong self-confidence, his mannerisms, his ego and his way of being able to continue to talk to you and get you to agree to his decision for the treatments or surgery.

I believed him when he continued to tell me I was just a very difficult case. After months that turned into years of physical therapy, taping, orthotics, braces, shots, and so much more. The possibility of conquering seemingly impossible odds kept getting harder and harder. I fought back with everything that I could give – physically, mentally, emotionally and spiritually.

The issues, problems and deception only continued to get worse. How could this possibly be happening?

Following the second surgery and the numerous questions that were left up in the air; especially with Dr. Hauser stating that he had no idea what could possibly be causing the continual spasms and unrelenting pain. Stating he had never seen anything like it before. I felt used and betrayed, and I was angry!

The experience of anger is normal and natural. As part of being made in God's image, humans have emotions, and one of those emotions is anger. Like all of God's gifts, anger has tremendous potential for good. We can choose to express our anger in ways that help or in ways that hinder, in ways that build or in ways that destroy. We can be irresponsible and allow the emotion of anger to control us, and we can express that anger in cruel and violent ways. Or, we can be wise by choosing to express our anger in healthy and positive ways.

It was a tremendous struggle. A further surgery by an amazing Orthopedic Foot & Ankle specialist to reconstruct my Posterior Tibial Tendon and to complete the Tarsal Tunnel Release that Dr. Hauser was unable to complete. It was during this time that I was formally diagnosed with a life changing condition called Complex Regional Pain Syndrome (CRPS). CRPS is believed to be caused by damage to, or malfunction of, the peripheral and central nervous systems. Currently, there is no cure. The best you can hope for is to put this disease into remission.

Mine is a story that so many chronic pain patients go through. The trials of traditional medicine, the lack of treatment options available to chronic pain patients, the lengths that patients are willing to go through to regain their lives, and the tremendous outcomes that can happen when you are willing to look outside the box.

This story is a true example of how I allowed God to heal my anger and then allowed Him to use my life's experience in making a difference in the lives of others living with chronic pain.

It is also a story of resilience, recovery, and a continuing desire to help others living with invisible illnesses and chronic pain.

INTRODUCTION

Pain is real and patients are searching for the solutions that will help them regain their lives. People of all ages are diagnosed with chronic pain every year. Pain does not discriminate. In the United States over 100 million people are diagnosed with some type of chronic pain.[1] This is greater than cancer, heart disease and diabetes combined.[2] However, pain reaches far past our borders and affects an astonishing 1.5 billion people worldwide.[3] Pain is a universal experience, serious and costly.

Chronic pain patients want to be heard and understood. Their pain is real, and they need solutions. They don't want to be told not to worry, that they don't look sick or that it's all in their head.

Everyone's story of how their pain began is unique, but there are common threads. There are times when we know what causes chronic pain and other times it's a mystery. Regardless, it's important for the individual to be heard, to find the help and resources they need that can help them regain function and regain their lives.

Pain is insidious and robs patients of even the smallest things in life. Perhaps someone is unable to work. Perhaps they can't do their shopping or laundry. Perhaps they can't play with their kids or be there for their spouse. For children it can keep them from school, sports, activities and their friends. This is where chronic pain affects people physically, mentally, emotionally, relationally and spiritually.

Most chronic pain patients see dozens of doctors and have had to perpetually re-tell their story, all the while feeling cross-examined about how many pills they are taking, even needing to bring them in to be randomly counted or to pee in a cup. They didn't get to this place on their own, and now they sit in a doctor's office with guarded hope.

Reflex Sympathetic Dystrophy Syndrome Association (RSDSA) estimates that there are about 50,000 new cases of CRPS a year in the United States. There is currently no tracking mechanism for how many people have been diagnosed across the world. CRPS is categorized as a rare disease and most physicians are not well versed in it.

Reflex Sympathetic Dystrophy (RSD), renamed as CRPS, is very much an unknown disease to the general public, because the symptoms do not make any sense when they're explained, and sometimes, the pain that's felt doesn't seem possible considering what you see is causing it. For instance, brushing a hand with a feather might cause significant pain for CRPS patients.

This is correct. I know this because I am one of those patients. I was diagnosed in 2007 with CRPS. It is a chronic neurological syndrome, and if you've never heard of it, you're not alone. But what you may not realize is how many people suffer from this condition.

- Mayo Clinic Study, which reported "an incidence rate of 5.46 per 100,000 person at risk, and a period prevalence of 20.57 per 100,000. Female:male ratio was 4:1, with a median age of 46 years at onset. Upper limb was affected twice as commonly as lower limb. All cases reported an antecedent event and fracture was the most common trigger (46%)."

- The McGill Pain Index was first developed in 1971 as a way of gauging the quality of pain. It was developed at McGill University by Melzack and Torgerson. According to McGill, person with a score of 0 effectively does not experience pain. A person with a high score, nearer to the highest score of 78, more than likely deals with chronic pain daily. CRPS suffers typically have pain that is in the range of 45 on an average day. The pain of CRPS is typically greater than what burn patients endure. This is real pain.

- For the majority of patients this condition starts in a limb. This can be foot, ankle, leg, hand or arm. It can start off from something as benign as an IV, an accident or following a surgery. According to the RSDSA organization.

  - According to the National Institute of Neurological Disorders and Stroke (NINDS), "In more than 90 percent of cases, the condition is triggered by a clear history of trauma or injury. The most common triggers are fractures, sprains/strains, soft tissue injury (such as burns, cuts, or bruises), limb immobilization (such as being in a cast), surgery, or even minor medical procedures such as needle stick."

  - It can occur in children as well. CRPS usually occurs following an injury.

From the onset of the condition, time is of the essence. The sooner the patient is diagnosed, and the sooner the treatments are started, the greater the odds are that the patient can regain their life and get into remission. At this time, there is no cure for CRPS. The best you can hope for is long-term remission, and that is currently the ultimate goal for anyone diagnosed.

There are two different types of Complex Regional Pain Syndrome: CRPS I – The symptoms of type I include: The presence of an initiating event such as a sprain. Continuing pain including allodynia, which is pain from a normal stimulus, such as the breeze from a ceiling fan, Hyperalgesia which an increased sense of pain to an unpleasant stimuli. The pain is disproportionate to that associated with the injury. There is edema (swelling), changes in skin (skin color changes, skin temperature changes), vasomotor changes, and excessive sweating in the region of pain.

CRPS II (Causalgia) – In Type II, a definite nerve injury can be identified. The symptoms are the same as in type I, but the cause is different. This is the presence of constant pain, allodynia (pain resulting from normal stimulus) or hyperalgesia (an increased sense of pain) after an identifiable nerve injury. There is still evidence of edema, and skin changes. This diagnosis is also one of exclusion based on the existence of conditions that would otherwise account for the degree of pain and dysfunction from a nerve injury.

The causes and the symptoms may vary a bit from person to person, but all those that suffer from CRPS have many things in common: they feel isolated, they feel like they are the only one going through this, and they just want the constant neuropathic pain to stop. Too often, they are afraid to admit it because of the stigma that still exists with chronic pain. That is how I felt until I finally realized that I could no longer continue living the way I was and sought out the help to get into remission - to get pain free and regain my life.

The day after I was notified my last spinal cord stimulator had caused a build-up of scar tissue on my dura, and that there was a possibility it could paralyze me, I scheduled the surgery to have it removed at a local hospital. Once the spinal cord stimulator was removed there would be no magic bullet – there isn't one for beating chronic pain, much less CRPS. Every doctor you speak with in the United States or anywhere in the world will tell you, "*There is no cure for CRPS.*" I was clearly told by my pain management doctor that he had run out of options and other than medication, opioids and NSAIDS, his options were nil. My research began for other treatment options just as quickly as the surgery was scheduled. Don't get me wrong when I make this statement, because the entire time I was diagnosed with CRPS I was continually looking for answers. This new challenge just put an immense burden on me, as the patient, to come up with the answer. I had a personal quest to fulfil, because once the spinal cord stimulator was removed, I was on my own. Day by day, hour by hour, minute by minute the time clicked by as I whittled down my options until I found my new starting point in my journey, my quest for a pain free life.

Now for the first time since I obtained remission or as I call it, *"regained my life"*, in 2013, I am publically sharing the intricate details of my struggle with CRPS, how I busted those chains and dug my way out of an ever growing sinkhole known as chronic pain – CRPS to be exact.

Other primary pieces of my journey that I will provide in this book are some of my personal journal entries I wrote during my journey, pictures from some of my treatments, but I am also including a resource section for patients, family members and caretakers. I want you to be able to see where I was with CRPS, the treatments that patients endure to get better, the healing process so that you can get a good grasp – and help erase some of the stigma – of chronic pain. You may be taken back by some pictures, or find some funny. This is real life dealing with CRPS or chronic pain. As I look back at where I was and where I am today, it was a life changing path.

I hope by sharing my journey it will help guide you on your journey or give you a better prospective on what a loved one is going through. If what I have gone through can assist you to help yourself as others have done for me then this book is worthwhile. If you have been pushing through CRPS, chronic pain, neuropathic pain, or any other invisible illness – you now need to take the next big step and take control of your future. It is not easy. It will take a lot of determination and hard work on your part. *But no matter what difficulties are in front of you, no matter how alone you feel, no matter how dark life may seem even when the sun is brightly shining, you can do it!* I have been where you are and I can tell you there is hope. I am living proof of it.

Never give up.

Names and identifying details have been changed to protect the privacy of individuals. This book is not intended as a substitute for the medical advice of physicians. The reader should regularly consult a physician in matters relating to his/her health and particularly with respect to any symptoms that may require diagnosis or medical attention.

CHAPTER 1

Taking the First Step

Like so many others, I sought out help from physicians, clinicians and others in the healthcare field. I was on a hunt to find relief, remission or a cure. But pain is often difficult to treat, requiring digging, advocating and a commitment to find solutions.

What so many don't understand is that pain is more than just an inconvenience; it encompasses the whole person. It affects how a person perceives their body's function and how they respond to the world. It affects us physically, mentally, emotionally, and spiritually. The loss is palpable.

Each of us has a turning point or a point in our lives where we have the *'ah ha'* moment.

It's that time where we realize that we can no longer go on living our lives the way we have, in the circumstances we have been living and something has to change. It's a moment in time caused by overwhelming pain, stress and aggravation of the lack of control over our situation, when we finally decide that something has to change. For some of us, depending on our personalities and the circumstances we're facing, it may take months or a few years to get to this point. For others, it could take decades. But indubitably, the intense frustration that we have allowed to swell up inside our minds and our bodies will eventually conquer all and push us to make a decision to search for the answers that await us.

The question is: will you grab hold of those answers as they are presented to you or will you stick with what you have been taught and not be open to new solutions? Sometimes you have to be willing to get on the life-raft when it is sent out to get you.

For me it took almost seven years of dealing with chronic pain and the debilitating condition of CRPS. That infamous day happened on a normally warm and sunny day in my home in Southern California. It was a beautiful day in the fall as is typical in Orange County; the sun shining bright through our Sycamore tree and a nice breeze was blowing in from the ocean. For me it was difficult to enjoy this time of year although in the past I had always looked forward to it. The damage that had been left behind from the CRPS was swift and wide spread. It was not only affecting my life it was affecting my entire family.

I had returned from a private clinic in Frankfurt, Germany a little over four weeks prior. When I returned my pain levels had dropped. I was functioning which was great and was just finishing up a regimen of a treatment that I brought home with me called "Regeneris". This is a custom mix of RNA cells meant to help my nerves regenerate. Recently my pain levels had started to incrementally ratchet back up in my foot, ankle, and throughout my back. The areas that were affected by the CRPS that had decreased while in Germany were starting to spread again. Why? I had already been treated at the clinic four times and every time I saw progress but in a matter of weeks it would rachet back up – every time. It just wasn't holding long-term.

Frustrated and feeling that I was running out of options I contacted the Medical Director in Germany again. We discussed my options: the possibility of returning to Frankfurt, doing another round of 'Regeneris', neural therapy, procaine IVs, etc…

At the same time that I was speaking with the Medical Director, I continued my ongoing search for any other options that may have opened up for other treatments of CRPS. I was on the internet, on the phone with former colleagues and researching anything that I could get my hands on. It would be nice for the treatment option to open up in the US, but at this point I was willing to go to the ends of the earth to get into remission… to get pain free.

What I did know was I could not go on living like this much longer. CRPS is a condition that causes a continual loop - your nerves are constantly receiving a signal from your brain that there is pain and/or trauma to a specific area of your body. The body is in fight and flight – sympathetic overload. For me I was in continual pain even with opioid pain medications. Lidocaine patches, Dilaudid, Methadone, Ketamine suspension, and other medications were not touching my pain. It was a never-ending cycle that went on 24/7 with no end in sight. On a daily basis my pain would range from a sharp burning pain, to throbbing and stabbing. There was no rhyme or reason, and no predicting this pain. Other times my lower left leg would turn a molten blue color and would feel cold like an ice cube, or it would turn red and be hot to the touch. CRPS not only affects the nerves, it also affects your vascular system, and as time goes on it can affect the immune system according to NINDS.

The slightest touch of anything, including a sheet on my skin caused intense pain, so I couldn't sleep with any covers on my foot or ankle. It didn't matter how cold it got. A gentle breeze, the air from a duct or fan would feel like a thousand needles being shoved through my skin. The pain was so intense that it was impossible for me to wear a sock on my left foot, much less a shoe. As my CRPS progressed into my back, from my waist to my shoulders that got tricky because the touch of a shirt caused intense pain yet you cannot run around naked.

It was imperative for me to find some answers. I had been praying for answers or for the correct treatment options to be put before me. I knew all along that I could not do this on my own and it was becoming even more apparent as time went on.

I received a message from a friend about a possible treatment in the US that may be an option. Then 24 hours later I received an email from another friend about a colleague of his that specialized in treating chronic pain patients and he, '...*highly suggested that I get in touch with them to see what I thought...*"

Honestly, I was intrigued and skeptical at the same time. How was this going to work when I had tried everything else? Yet, in my heart I knew that I could not leave one stone unturned and there was an old saying, "*I would spit on a spark plug if I knew it would work...*"

I contacted their office and I did my best to gather information about the type of patients they had treated, outcomes, long-term success, and any other question I could come up with. We also discussed my history with CRPS, where I was, where I wanted to go and what my goals were. This was a very intriguing concept to me especially because I had tried hypnosis early on in my diagnosis to no avail. Yet this was different. This was based on the biology and physiology of the body, the brain, neuroplasticity and clinical hypnosis. This was completely different than anything I had tried before and the theory actually made sense.

The other options could include high dose Ketamine infusions. I had previously contacted a doctor in Florida about this procedure and there were a lot of unanswered questions with regard to CRPS and outcomes. I had already been on an oral Ketamine suspension for years. The infusions are a big step, but the problem is that they do not last long-term. At the time most high dose Ketamine infusions were done in an ICU in a hospital for three days for the initial infusions, and now they are doing them in out-patient centers or even physician offices. Most patients need to have what they call 'Ketamine boosts' to stay pain free or in remission every 3-6 months. The big question I asked with the infusions was, "...*were there any studies on any potential long-term side effects of that high of a dosage of ketamine?*" I was told that at that time there were no long-term studies available. On a personal note, for me, that was a bit scary and I didn't want to take that risk.

Now the majority of the physician are doing Ketamine Infusions on an out-patient basis.

I also looked into another treatment protocol that was fairly new at the time called Calmare aka Scrambler Therapy. The Calmare device uses a biophysical rather than a biochemical approach. A 'no-pain' message is transmitted to the nerves via disposable surface electrodes applied to the skin in the region of the patient's pain. The perception of pain is cancelled when the no-pain message replaces that of pain, by using the same pathway through the surface electrodes in a non-invasive way. They had just started utilizing Calmare on CRPS patients and had very little data available to give me on outcomes. This was a little bothersome. Plus, they kept impressing on me that the maximum benefit would be achieved through follow-up treatments. Meaning, patients would have to return for 'boost' treatments periodically as needed depending on the severity of their CRPS. I wanted a treatment that could legitimately get me into remission and keep me pain free long-term without worrying about continual treatments.

I needed and wanted something that was proven, a treatment protocol that could help me over the long-term.

The clock was ticking, my pain was getting worse and a decision had to be made. No one could make this decision for me. My mind was spinning as every possible scenario was running through it and I was reflecting back on what brought me to this point.

CHAPTER 2

Sprain to Pain

A sprained ankle, how could an innocuous sprained ankle turn into a diagnosis of *'plantar fasciitis'*, and then insurmountable pain? Hindsight being 20/20 it probably wasn't the case, but you know the old saying, *"If I only knew then, what I know now..."*

At the most basic level, pain plays a protective role in our lives and is a normal response to an injury or disease. Without the alarm system of pain, none of us would survive. It is when that alarm signal persists that pain becomes a chronic problem.

Early 2006 I was referred to a local Podiatric surgeon, Dr. Hauser, since my sprained ankle wasn't healing properly. He seemed nice enough at the time. Good bedside manner, courteous, and started off with a conservative treatment plan of physical therapy, getting arch supports and a C.A.M. (controlled ankle movement) boot. I followed his protocol as prescribed and my pain continued to get worse around my posterior tibial tendon. This was several months after Hurricane Katrina tore through New Orleans, and I had already planned and coordinated an outreach team to head back to New Orleans. It was much more than a typical rebuilding trip. I was the leader of a volunteer group called Young Life working with emancipated young adults from the foster care system. This was their opportunity to give back, to give of themselves and to put themselves out there like they had never done before, and they were all looking forward to this trip. They had followed the news, seen the destruction and it struck a chord with them. This was a rebuilding trip for both those in New Orleans and for the inner workings of these young adults. I had to make this trip! I was their leader and I was the only female leader going on this trip. I had enlisted some male volunteer leaders to go with me, but I had many other young ladies going on the trip so if I didn't go they - didn't go.

As the trip got closer my left ankle and foot were just not getting better. The physical therapy was not helping; cortisone shots made no difference and the CAM boot seemed to be making things worse.

On my next visit to Dr. Hauser I told him that I had to make this trip and I tried to explain how important it was for the group that I was involved with. Needless to say he was none too happy with me. After several terse looks and some chastising, a plan was devised where we both felt fairly confident that I could make this trip safely. He wrote me additional scripts for pain medications and NSAIDS, he told me to make sure I had proper boots to wear, etc... Last but not least to make sure to contact him upon returning to let him know how I was doing and to set up a follow-up appointment.

I was excited but leery at the same time. Planning for this trip had been going on for quite some time, I had received grant money to cover the trip for the group and had everything set up. Yet, I knew that my ankle was not steady and it would be a constant uphill battle the entire trip.

It was time to reach down and dig deep as I had talked to this group about many times. The CAM boot came off and a light brace went on. I packed plenty of disposable ice packs, ace-bandages, NSAIDS and filled my prescriptions. These would be essential to getting me through this trip.

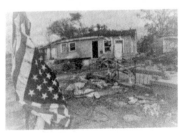

Upon return my ankle pain was intense. It was the medial ankle or inside of my ankle as I had rolled it when I injured it initially. I contacted Dr. Hauser the following business day after arriving back from New Orleans and he was still in disbelief that I made the trip.

We met in his office to reassess the condition of my left ankle and foot following my return. Physical Therapy has not helped, cortisone injections were not helping and the CAM boot was just hindering the situation. Additional X-Rays were taken and I was told that I needed surgery to release my plantar fascia. Once that was done it would relieve the pain and I would be back on my feet in a matter of weeks.

Well, if it was that easy then of course I was willing to do an outpatient surgery to take care of it. It seemed like an easy enough procedure and the recovery would be a slam dunk.
The surgery was scheduled two weeks later at an outpatient surgery center.

CHAPTER 3

Surgeries

Was a diagnosis of Plantar Fasciitis really what was causing my pain? The conservative treatments haven't worked up to this point and I needed to try something to make the sprained ankle get better, so if this is it then let's do it.

I was told that it was a 'minor' outpatient procedure and should be walking by the next day. Well, that changed along the way. It was an outpatient surgery, it took a little longer than anticipated, I left on crutches, NWB (non-weight bearing) and back in a lovely new CAM boot.

How was this progress?

Needless to say, I was not the typical Plantar Fasciitis release patient, as I was told. I was kept on crutches and sent back to physical therapy. If I wasn't on my foot it was ok, but as soon as I put pressure on my foot or had it in specific positions it became painful. The pain was always in a very defined area.

I continued with the rehabilitation as prescribed

following my outpatient surgery. Yet, days turned into weeks, and weeks turned into months with no resolution. My left foot and ankle were just not getting any better.

I returned over and over to my doctor's office and was told I needed to have patience. My patience was running thin and things were just not getting better.

Finally, a MRI was ordered and I was told that I had an 'Accessory Navicular'. This in layman's terms is an extra bone in your foot. The thought process was that the Accessory Navicular was larger than normal and was putting pressure on the surrounding structures causing pain.

Resolution: to surgically remove the Accessory Navicular from the left foot.

It was explained that is was a fairly routine surgery, I would be NWB (non-weight bearing) for 4-6 weeks following the surgery and then would require more physical therapy. It seemed pretty straight forward to both myself and my family.

I did my due diligence and looked it up on the internet, talked to some colleagues about the procedure and it seemed like it was a clear cut surgery. If this was the final step to taking away my foot pain then of course I was willing to do it. I could manage 4-6 weeks on crutches again, so I scheduled the surgery with Dr. Hauser.

All my pre-op labs were done and the next morning was the big day. I knew the routine all too well. Nothing to eat or drink after midnight, etc.

The following morning we got up at the crack of dawn to head off to the surgery center. My stomach was in knots. I always played it off like I was cool as a cucumber for my family, but this morning I was just uneasy and nervous.

The second hand on the clock on the wall above the check-in seemed to click slower and slower with each passing minute. Why was this time any different than my previous surgeries? I just kept telling myself this was ridiculous.

When I was called back I was a "nervous Nellie" this time. Perhaps I should have listened to my instincts. One never knows.

This morning I was taken back for my surgery and as usual the Versed given to me in the pre-op area did nothing and I was wheeled back watching the scenery. They are not used to a patient going into the OR completely with it when they are still trying to prep the OR and the OR Techs are running around. As a matter of fact it makes them rather uncomfortable. They couldn't ask the anesthesiologist to work any faster.

What I would find out afterwards was - this was no normal surgery. Somehow, some where, for some unknown reason this took a very drastic turn for the worse. What should have been a routine surgery to remove an accessory navicular turned out to be the first step down the very slippery slope of CRPS due to several errors that were made during my surgery. My posterior tendon was ruptured, a 4-5 cm gap was left in it so that they could not just reconnect it on its own, etc. They used a cadaver allograft to reconnect my posterior tendon.

When I awoke from this surgery I was in immense pain, I was shocked to hear they had to use a cadaver allograft to reattach my posterior tendon and my little toe was spasming, also known as dystonia. Dr. Hauser had absolutely no idea what to do other than to try to reassure me that things would be ok and that I just needed time to heal.

The day of my surgery Dr. Hauser left on vacation and left me in the hands of his colleague. His partner and colleague had the pleasure of taking my calls that afternoon when my pain was out of control, later that evening and the following day. I ended up unwrapping my foot per doctor's orders to check the incision to find it red and inflamed following the surgery. We had no idea if my body was rejecting the allograft, if I was having an allergic reaction, if there was an infection starting, or if it was something else.

By the following day, Saturday, I ended up at the ER due to pain and the redness that continued to spread. Both my family and I were furious that we were unable to reach the on-call doctor considering I was 24 hours post-op and this was a huge deal that should not have happened. The attending physician in the ER was in awe that the surgeon and his partner were not responding to calls and did their best to reassure us. A line was drawn around the redness so we could gauge if it was getting worse, I was given antibiotics and sent on my way.

I ended up leaving several messages through the exchange for both my surgeon and his partner about the situation and lack of response.

Unfortunately, the redness and pain continued. I was in the doctor's office the next business day on an emergent basis. He could not believe what my foot and ankle looked like. He tried to break the ice a bit with asking if I was, "*Ms. Louisiana*" and laughing. I wasn't thinking clearing and wasn't putting the pieces together at the moment, but the more he spoke I found out Dr. Hauser was in his office the day I called after returning from New Orleans. He laughed as he filled me in on their conversation.

A culture of the area was taken, different antibiotics were prescribed and a topical medication was applied. I was to follow-up with him to see if there was any relief while waiting for the test results and my surgeon to return.

During this time I was also seen my by neurologist

and she was beside herself when she saw my foot. Horrified would be a good definition of her response. She was ready to send me to an Infectious Disease specialist or anyone that could get a handle on what was happening. We agreed to give it another week to see if it settled down on its own.

Eventually the redness went away but the pain did not. I was never given a copy of the culture to see what came of it. My little toe on my left foot continued to spasm 24 hours a day. It didn't matter if I was sleeping or awake.

I was sent to different Neurologists per the request of my podiatrist. I had EMG testing completed. No one could figure out what to do to stop the continual spasm. I was offered such things as Botox, but the reality was they were guessing whether it would even work.

My trust was beginning to wane to say the least at this point. There is an old saying that talks about, "the practice of medicine", and I definitely felt like I was the one being used for practice.

CHAPTER 4

Searching for Answers

It's difficult to overstate the extent to which pain can disrupt a person's life. While for some, pain represents a persistent, annoying distraction that interrupts the flow of the day, others find it decreases their capacity to function. Pain may affect walking or doing physical activities people once enjoyed, thus affecting overall well-being. The extra effort required to do normal things becomes fatiguing, so there is less energy and incentive to do once-enjoyable activities.

When pain becomes chronic, it invades our relationships, finances, identity and more. It tries to overtake our lives and will succeed if we allow it to. It can be persistent. Pain, when persistent, creates distress and impairment that can negatively impact quality of life.

Chronic pain forces us to stop, to take inventory, and to focus on what is valuable in our lives. We learn to be our own best advocate and to search for the answers and treatment options that can help us regain our lives.

My search began. I wasn't comfortable with the answers I was given. My foot and ankle were worse than they were after my sprain, and now my little toe was in continual spasms. I knew something was dreadfully wrong as my pain levels continued to increase.

I was referred to a highly regarded Orthopedic Foot and Ankle surgeon to get a second opinion. I brought all of my OP reports, X-rays and MRI reports. I was so hopeful that he would hold the answers and allow me to regain what was continuing to slip away.

The moment of reckoning was there. I felt I was finally going to get my answers. My visit was thorough but heart breaking. Based upon my exam, previous OP reports and test results it was determined that a Tarsal Tunnel Release could provide me with the relief I needed and was seeking. One huge problem. There were many inconsistencies in my OP reports that were throwing out red flags. These red flag posed problems that the new doctor felt were errors. Thus, I was told he didn't want to get involved in a '*complicated*' case. The complicated had nothing to do with the surgery that needed to be done. Instead the complicated had to do with the possible surgical errors made in the previous surgery, not knowing if there could be any legal action taken, etc. It didn't matter what I said he was walking away, and I felt that I was being discarded.

I left his office that day feeling abandoned. If a surgeon made an error and another highly regarded surgeon does not want to fix the situation – where does this leave the patient? Where did it leave me?

A follow-up appointment was set with my neurologist who knew the orthopedic surgeon I had met with. She was beside herself and in disbelief that he would not take my case. She understood the gravity of my situation. She knew that I needed a competent surgeon and I needed help. At the same time she had a hard time understanding why I would be held responsible for the errors of a podiatrist when something needed to be done. She couldn't sit by idly so she placed a call to the orthopedic surgeon. Unfortunately, she received a very similar response to what I received in his office.

Next stop was back to my primary care physician. I brought my medical records, OP reports, and test results. I explained my predicament to her and asked her what she would do if she were in my situation. She was very understanding of my situation and we decided that I should try to get another opinion from a top rated podiatrist.

Finally, the day came to see the new podiatrist for another opinion. I had this down by now. Medical records, OP reports and tests were all taken in for review. He was taken back by my little toe and the continual rhythmical movement (i.e. spasms aka dystonia). A quick exam was completed.

Again there were some raised eyebrows with my OP reports. I was told that a 'Tarsal Tunnel Release' may be a possible solution but he would feel better about having the orthopedic surgeon do it based on the previous surgeries to my foot and ankle. He knew the orthopedic surgeon I had just consulted with and knew he had an excellent reputation. It was suggested that I see if he would reconsider. If he wouldn't then, "... *please return and we will look at your options*." Well, this is not a very promising thing to hear.

Walking from the office my mind wouldn't turn off. Frustration, anger, sadness, animosity – you name it I was feeling it. How could this be happening? How can I be put in a spot where I cannot get the help I need to fix a problem caused by a surgeon who made an error? How is this fair?

My frustrations were continuing to grow. This was the first time that I sincerely felt that the medical community as a whole was letting me down. My hope and faith that I would find a resolution was beginning to waiver.

Back to my primary care physician. The anticipation sitting in the exam room waiting for her was horrific. I had a million thoughts going through my head, my stress was through the roof, and the worst part was I knew that she had personally seen the initial podiatric surgeon. The minutes waiting seemed like hours as my anticipation was enormous.

Dr. Hamelet arrived, observed my left foot/ankle, said she didn't want to examine me as she knew it would be too painful, and we went over the events since I last saw her. She was very frustrated but not surprised that I was having difficulty getting another surgeon to step into my case. As she put it, "... *your case is very complicated and most surgeons are not going to want to get involved.*" We continued the conversation and discussed what I had been told about possible surgical errors that could have caused what I was currently dealing with. She looked at the floor and shook her head. I know she knew what I was told was correct, but she had a hard time admitting it because as she had previously told me she knew the podiatrist that did the surgeries.

I finally asked her, "*If this were a family member or even you what would you do?*" She thought for a minute, and reiterated that she had referred family members to Dr. Hauser and had personally been treated by him. She followed this with, "...*I think he is the only surgeon that will know what was done in the area. He will know where he went and what needs to be done.*" I questioned this comment based upon what I had been told by the two prior surgeons, but Dr. Hamelet reiterated that she felt he would do a good job at a Tarsal Tunnel Release and she would go back to him.

Once again, I felt like I was on my own when I left her office. I had tried unsuccessfully to get an orthopedic surgeon and a top podiatrist to intercede. Now, I am being told to return to the surgeon that left me in this mess. Wow!

I returned to my neurologist and we discussed what Dr. Hamelet had to say. On one hand she could see where she was coming from and on the other hand she was a little concerned and would much prefer the orthopedic surgeon to be involved. She examined my foot and ankle again. The pain was not getting any better. This time she mentioned something that we had not discussed before and that was a 'possible diagnosis' of CRPS. She said she had other patients with the condition and I was starting to fall into the category, but she wasn't ready to hit me with this diagnosis yet. She was hopeful that the Tarsal Tunnel Release would resolve the nerve pain and that everything would be ok. Yet, she did ask me to talk to Dr. Hauser about this possibility.

CHAPTER 5

Return to the Scene

With a deep pit and butterflies forming in the middle of my stomach I returned to Dr. Hauser's office for a consultation. I wasn't ready to commit to him doing another surgery, but I did want to get his input since no one else would touch my case with a ten-foot-pole. Honestly, I felt like I was between a rock and a hard spot with very few options.

As I sat there waiting for him in the very familiar room I could feel my face becoming flush and my stress levels rising. I felt like I had half of me asking what the heck I was doing back in this office, and then I had the other half of me saying that if he couldn't fix the issues he caused then I was totally screwed.

The normal knock on the door and then comes in Dr. Hauser with the smile, exuding confidence, good bedside manner, and charisma. I was very upfront with him and explained that I had sought out two other opinions about the condition of my foot and ankle. He sat there very attentive listening to what I had to say and wanted to know how they felt it should be handled. I didn't disclose who I sought out, but I did disclose that both had agreed that a Tarsal Tunnel Release could be the best option to helping with the pain. They both felt there was an entrapment of the nerve(s) and by doing a release it could stop or minimize the pain I was currently dealing with. Neither surgeon knew what to do with my little toe nor how to get the spasm to stop, but the main concern was the constant pain. I then brought up the possible question of CRPS by my Neurologist, and he quickly dismissed it.

Dr. Hauser examined my foot and ankle. He agreed that based on the current situation that a Tarsal Tunnel Release (TTR) would be the best solution. He wanted to try to block the lateral plantar nerve to the toe to see if he could get it to stop moving. He requested to do one or two injections to block the nerve. I agreed as it could be done there in his office.

I moved over to the procedure room so that he could have access to Marcaine and the appropriate syringes. I thought I was going to pass out with the first injection. The pain was immense and once he completed the injection he said I shouldn't feel anything. Well, that just wasn't the case. My fifth toe was moving even quicker and the pain was more intense than prior to the injection. Dr. Hauser had me wait a few minutes and kept saying that it should have blocked the nerve and made the area numb, but it did neither. He insisted on doing a second injection. Same results – nothing but increased pain. I could see the frustration on his face. I was doing the best I could to breathe through the pain and to try to concentrate on anything else in the room. This continued as he was on a mission to try to block this area. Five injections later I had a puppet brigade going with my fifth through second toes as they were all moving in tandem. Plus, I was in more pain than when I walked through his door. I finally said I couldn't take any more injections and we were reaching the maximum amount of Marcaine that could safely be injected into an area.

Following my appointment I had a lot of thinking to do. I talked to friends, family, colleagues and a couple other doctors about the situation too. Everyone came to an agreement that something had to be done and if Dr. Hauser was my only option then I would need to move forward.

Many prayers were said from many different areas both locally and throughout the world for a safe surgery and a good outcome.

The morning finally arrived. When we made it to the surgery center my stomach was in knots, millions of butterflies, and my head had tons of thoughts going through it. I just felt uneasy but I kept telling myself it would be ok. The history of this surgery center, the familiar smells, familiar sights, and the not so great outcomes were just flooding through me. I couldn't stop them.

I glanced at the clock; each passing minute seemed like an hour. Finally, I was called back to the all too familiar area with gurneys lined up, IV poles waiting to be utilized, and the hospital gown waiting. I put on the stoic face and continued on, as it wasn't my first rodeo. The nurses commented on how I looked so familiar and I sarcastically responded that I was a, "*frequent flier.*"

Dr. Hauser was quick to come out to the pre-op holding area. He ultimately held the keys to my happiness and my health in his hands. I felt helpless at that moment in time. He tried to assure me that everything would be fine and instructed the nursed to push Versed while I was waiting as he knew I was anxious and stressed out. As usual the Versed given to me in the pre-op area did nothing and I was wheeled back watching the scenery.

The staff was still prepping the OR when I arrived. Music playing, staff scurrying and people looking at me like why are you so wide awake. I really didn't want to be aware of what they were doing at that time. Once moved from the gurney to the OR table I had a quick conversation with my anesthesiologist and then I was out for the count.

Groggy but starting to come around my pain was immense. I remember a nurse asking if I was in pain and responding, yes. Then I was out again. When I started to come back around the nurse was asking about pain levels and had a lot of questions. The big thing she wanted to know was if my little toe was moving. I could feel my little toe moving, pressing on the side of the dressing every time it moved, and my pain levels were not good. I asked if Dr. Hauser was still there and they said, no, but he left orders to call him. Before I knew it I had a phone being given to me and being told that Dr. Hauser wanted to speak to me. This was a first. Plus, I was not exactly with it. He tried to tell me that the surgery went well and when they finished my little toe was not moving. I told him that my little toe was still moving and that my pain levels were not controlled. He assured me that once the swelling went down everything would be fine. But, just before hanging up he mentioned that there was a problem with the posterior tibial tendon (PTT), but not to worry about it. He'd talk to me in the office.

Did I hear that correctly?!? What happened this time? I was groggy, in pain and the surgery center was trying to get me out of there because I was the last patient.

On the way home my family tried to explain to

me that the posterior tibial tendon was ruptured. They were told it was not in the surgical field and that the surgeon opted to focus on the Tarsal Tunnel Release rather than also repairing the PTT. Was I really hearing this correctly? I was furious to say the least.

Waiting for my post-op visit to arrive was nerve racking. I spoke with my neurologist and a couple other physicians and everyone said the same thing, *"He should have taken the time to have repaired the Posterior Tibial Tendon prior to closing the surgery. The risk of having a patient go through a secondary surgery far surpasses any risk of extending a surgery to complete it 100%..."* This input only reinforced my feelings that Dr. Hauser was completely over his head.

My first post-op visit was full of anticipation, frustration and questions. My family had been told by Dr. Hauser that my Posterior Tibial Tendon (PTT) had ruptured, but he felt it was more important to tend to the Tarsal Tunnel Release. He stated the PTT could be repaired later if needed. I was absolutely speechless. I wanted to verify with Dr. Hauser directly if this was indeed the case and why the heck would he not have repaired the PTT since it helps propel you forward when you walk. This is a vital part of your foot integrity, the ankle, provides stability and is essential. It was quite the conversation as he backed up his decision and held his ground that he did what he felt was in my best interest at the time. There was zero reasoning with him and what was done was done.

The pain did not decrease in the days and weeks following the surgery and my fifth toe did not stop moving. As a matter of fact my pain was worse!

Dr. Hauser did his obligatory post op visits with me, but he honestly had no answers for the pain or why my toe was still spasming.

He declined having me return to physical therapy as he felt that could compromise the release. Instead he wanted me to do passive range of motion exercises at home and to continue in a CAM boot.

CHAPTER 6

Pulling Strings

Uncertainty and a lack of understanding about what was occurring in my body could have made it easy for me to lose hope. But with the encouragement of my family, friends, and my neurologist and through the depth and strength of my faith I knew I had to continue my search for answers. I didn't want to live in fear.

Hope and despair are two opposing emotions, and there can be a struggle between them. All the moments of pain in our day to day living can lead to hope or despair. Hope requires action and directional movement towards the future. It is not static. Hope focuses on recovery. It's seeing threads of light in a dark tunnel. Despair is shaped by pain, limitations, dependency, worry and fear. Hopelessness is the end result of despair. It is the end of the process of giving up and losing a future perspective.

When you are dealing with chronic pain, the feelings of hope and despair can alternate. Hope may be present at the beginning and then wane as time goes by. If you give in completely to despair, you arrive at hopelessness. But if you hold on to hope, you can survive and even thrive during the most difficult days.

I was trying to hold onto hope as the weeks and months of post-op appointments had put me back at my neurologist's office. It was both a follow-up visit and a fact-finding mission. My fifth toe (small toe) was still spasming and my pain levels were crazy. It was a sharp, burning pain that was different than the typical post-op pain that I had experienced in the past. I was holding onto hope that my neurologist could help me find some answers.

I had brought a copy of my OP report from the Tarsal Tunnel Release (TTR) and many questions. She was thorough as usual with going over the OP report and doing an exam on my foot and ankle. The exam had me cringing and holding tight due to the pain that I was experiencing.

Once again questions were raised about CRPS, but she said it could be post-op pain due to the TTR. She wanted to start me on medication just in case it was CRPS, but was not ready to say that was the culprit of the pain.

She was adamant about having me do another consult with the orthopedic surgeon. I just laughed and said that would not happen especially since he flatly turned me away and said he didn't want to get involved in my case. She saw the despair in my face and knew that the situation was spiraling out of control. She excused herself and came back in with her personal cell phone. The next thing I knew she had the orthopedic surgeon on the phone discussing my case and telling him that if he wasn't willing to get involved that no one would. She pulled the colleague and friend cards to try to pull all the strings necessary to get me back through his door.

It worked!

The following week I had a return appointment to the orthopedic foot and ankle surgeon. I brought with me the new OP report and any new test results.

Although I dreaded this appointment, I also had hope that there could be something done to help alleviate the situation. This surgeon was one of the best in the area of foot and ankle reconstruction and he was an instructor at a top teaching university.

The knock on the door, the confident blonde haired ortho coming in and matter of fact answers being put forth. This was a cut to the chase type of an appointment. He clearly remembered me and my case. Flatly stating he didn't need to exam my foot or ankle as he had reviewed the OP reports and knew what was done. He pointed out the incision from the TTR and commented that it was not where an incision would be placed for a proper release. Based upon the incision area he had no idea how much damage had been done, but he knew that it was not possible to completely release the nerves from that angle. He was staunch that the Posterior Tibial Tendon did need to be reconstructed, but he had no idea what it would take based upon the previous surgeries and things that had occurred. Our conversation continued and he agreed to schedule the needed surgery.

A couple days prior to the surgery I met with the anesthesiologist to discuss my case, the possible diagnosis of CRPS and what could be done to contain it if it was indeed CRPS. He agreed to do an additional block just below the knee and to utilize Ketamine during the surgery. He had worked with other patients that had neuropathic pain and CRPS.

The day of the surgery I was a bit anxious, but I was also excited at the very real possibility that this could be the end of an arduous adventure. Dr. Michael, my orthopedic surgeon, came in with a resident. He was confident, prepped and ready for the surgery. Next in was my anesthesiologist. He was great. He wheeled me back to the OR to start prepping me for the surgery. This was the first time I had ever had Ketamine prior and during a surgery and I will say that it was quite the flight. I remember seeing bright vivid images and feeling like the room was spinning for a short time.

Post-op was ready to take on the challenge of my case. The nurses were great and making sure my pain was in check. Dr. Michael stopped by my bed-side to talk with me and I could see him charting in the corner of the room while I was in recovery too. That was quite the change from my other surgeries with my podiatrist. Things were a bit fuzzy at the time, but I knew I would be filled in later that day when I got home.

I was told that they had to harvest a tendon from my foot to reconstruct the Posterior Tibial Tendon, the Tarsal Tunnel Release was successful, but Dr. Michael was not sure what was going to happen with my fifth toe. He said it looked like a bomb went off in my foot. It was a mess.

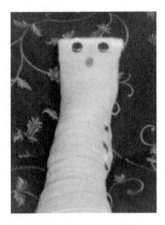

I returned to Dr. Michael's office just a few days after my surgery to remove the soft dressing and to be put into a cast. My foot and ankle were still a bit swollen and it was very sensitive to the touch. No one seemed concerned about this. Prior to the cast being put on the tech cleaned the area and applied some steri-strips to the area over the stitches to make sure everything would be secure. I picked out the color of my cast and we were off and running.

Within 24 hours something was wrong. My pain levels were increasing and it was just unmanageable. I contacted Dr. Michael's office and was asked to come in to get the cast checked. They decided to remove it. The vibration of cutting it off was incredibly painful. The tech kept looking at me like I was crazy and kept telling me that they could not cut me. They thought I was just being overly sensitive and that I was worried about having the cast taken off. Unfortunately, this was not the case. When it was taken off the area around the incision and steri-strips were red and had some blisters. I was allergic to the steri-strips. Therefore they had to be taken off. Each one that was peeled off felt like they were taking my skin with it. I couldn't explain the pain and in my head it made absolutely no sense. Then another cast was put on.

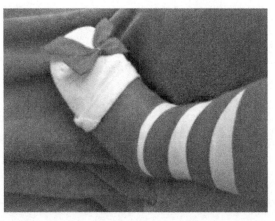

Approximately 2 weeks later it was time for the cast to be removed and for the stitches to come out. This should have been a happy, jump for joy time. Instead it was the most painful experience. Again, the tech could not understand why removing stitches could be so painful. I just about hit the roof with the first one that was removed. The tech knew he had to finish and said he would be as careful as possible and kept apologizing along the way. I was sweating profusely, ready to puke and pale white by the time they were done. They couldn't get Dr. Michael in the room quick enough.

He still didn't want to confirm nor deny a diagnosis of CRPS.

CHAPTER 7

Diagnosis

A personal referral from my neurologist over to Dr. Amir was initiated. He was a highly regarded pain management doctor, associate professor and someone that was familiar with CRPS. It took a few weeks to get in which seemed like an eternity.

I was a bundle of nerves that morning while waiting to meet Dr. Amir. On one hand I felt like I really needed to know if I indeed had CRPS, but on the other hand I was scared to death. This was the first time I had ever been to a Pain Management doctor and I wondered if this was where I really belonged as I looked around at the other patients waiting. Was I really as bad off as the others sitting here? Was this what I had to look forward to? My heart started to pound the more I thought about it.

My name was called as the door opened to the back area. There was very little talk as I was roomed. I immediately sat in the chair instead of sitting on the exam table. I just couldn't bring myself to do that yet. I was told that Dr. Amir would be with me in just a few minutes.

It seemed like time was standing still as the minutes clicked by. I finally heard the slight knock on the door and then saw Dr. Amir enter the room. He came in and introduced himself. I had brought him the normal dump of medical records, OP reports, etc. He had them in his file, but said he would prefer to hear from me what was happening, then he would complete an exam and let me know what he thought. That seemed fair and started to clear the air. At least he was willing to listen.

As I went over everything that had happened over the past year and a half, I could see his mind clicking. He was taking notes and observing my foot, toe and ankle in between. He was actually paying attention.

I felt apprehensive as he pulled his stool over to take a closer look at my foot and ankle. He could tell that I was nervous for him to touch my lower leg as it was extremely hypersensitive. He assured me that it would be ok. He had me place my foot and ankle on his leg so that he could take a closer look. Then he gently touched different areas to see how sensitive it was and where the sensitivity ended. He was looking at the coloration and any vascular changes. He was really paying attention to my little toe that wouldn't stop moving the entire visit. The more time he took with me the more confident I was that he was coming to his own conclusion rather than pulling a conclusion from my medical records.

With a very matter of fact tone, Dr. Amir, said he had good news and bad news. I was anxious for answers, but the last thing I wanted was more bad news.

Bad news was he diagnosed me with CRPS. Good news was he felt it was caught early enough that we could get it into remission. He said it would need to be treated aggressively, but he was confident we could get a handle on it in six months to a year.

I had many questions and Dr. Amir took the time to answer them to the best of his ability. A few things that were said still stand out today.

"This is serious."
"There is no cure for CRPS."
"Yes, it can and will change your life..."

He wanted to change my medications and to start with some local and regional blocks to see if that would help. It was the hope that he put out there that allowed me to keep going at that point.

I left his office that day wondering what was in front of me. I felt like I still had a million questions. My pain was validated with a definitive diagnosis, but I was not ready for a diagnosis that didn't have a cure. Driving home I felt as though I was in a fog.

◆ ◆ ◆

Once home I did what most people would do that received a diagnosis that they were not 100% sure what it meant - I went online. That may have been the worst mistake I had made yet. The articles, pictures and stories were horrific and scared the hell out of me.

How could anything be this bad? The stories were gloom and doom. There was nothing, and I mean absolutely not one shred of positive that I could find out there on CPRS or outcomes.

I emailed some friends in the medical field and jumped online to a group a doctors that I knew. When I started asking about CRPS I was immediately asked if I was diagnosed with it. *Yes, I was*. One doctor replied with, "... *unfortunately, Traci, life as you know it will end...*" Really? I knew my pain was bad, but how much worse could it possibly get?

I finally sought out a couple of online support groups but they were not a huge help either. The majority of the information posted in the groups consisted of people venting on how bad they were doing, how life was horrific, about treatments that were not working, and thoughts of suicide. Don't get me wrong... I am glad there was a place where people could vent. On the other hand I didn't feel that was the support that I was looking for or that I needed.

CHAPTER 8

When Pain Doesn't Stop

Now that I had taken inventory and was trying to wrap my head around a definitive diagnosis, it was just as important for me to understand the science of the pain. Knowing how pain works in the body can help us understand how complex chronic pain originates and why it can be so difficult to manage. This can also give us an advantage over pain and the pathways in which it travels within the body. I'm sharing this with you as it took me years to figure this out. The more we understand, the more effective you can make changes.

The key idea to understand is that for optimal control of pain, we need to access and control pain pathways in our body in as many strategic places as we can.

Pain Pathways

When tissue injury occurs in the body, it activates a process called nociception. Information about the injury travels to small nerve fibers in the spinal cord. Sometimes the body responds reflexively to this information, such as when you with-draw your hand from a hot fire or jerk back when you step on a sharp object.

Other times that information travels up to the brain, which assigns to that message the sensation of pain. The feeling of pain is not registered in the body but rather in the brain. Here pain is assigned its location within the body, the type and sever-ity of the injury is assessed, and the context in which the event occurred is recorded. Emotions are attached to pain as well. All of this happens to create a learning process by which we understand something is dangerous – and we try to avoid it in the future. Thus, the nociception pathways and the sensation of pain within the brain work to-gether as a protective mechanism to prevent fur-ther injury.

The experience and the sensation of pain occur in the context of our lives and our histories. The protective process partly explains why the perception of pain varies greatly from person to person. Pain perception can also change within an individual over time. This is why emotions, expectations, perspectives and attitudes can con-tribute to one's pain level. In short, there can be strong emotions and upsetting memories at-tached to pain that may need to be addressed too.

Nociceptive pathways are much like a complex highway system. They have multiple lanes, on and off ramps, forks in the road, times of increased activity, gates that might open or close, and even traffic cops that direct a nociceptive message along the way before it reaches the brain. If multiple gates along the highway are switched open, that message gets sent to the brain to be interpreted as pain.

In the 1960's, Ronald Melzack, a Canadian psychologist, and David Wall, a British neuroscientist, proposed the gate control theory of pain, which, though our understanding continues to evolve, has been generally accepted by the scientific community as how we process noxious information in the body and recognize it as pain in the brain.

As already mentioned, when an injury occurs, information about the injury is transmitted from the injured tissue to the spinal cord and then travels up to the brain. However, along this pathway, the signal encounters nerve gates and must pass through these gates in order to reach the brain. These nerve gates are actually different type of nerves called neuromodulators. These nerve gates function to reduce or stop the nociceptive signal to keep it from reaching the brain, where it is recognized as pain. If the activity on the pathway to the brain is strong or persistent enough to overwhelm the gates, the gates are opened, and when the signal reaches the brain, it is sensed as pain. Sometimes these gates are open long after the offending stimulus is removed, or the injured part of the body has healed. The pathway can also develop a maladaptive response, and the message is either always being transmitted or is transmitted more easily. In other words, it is like the pain message pathway is always switched on or more easily switched on. This process is called sensitization.

At the root of this process of sensitization is neuroplasticity. Neuroplasticity refers to adaptive changes within the brain and central nervous system. The brain can learn and adapt to new things. For instance, when a person learns to ride a bike, new connections are made within the brain and become reinforced and more efficient with practice. Eventually, we are riding our bike without training wheels, and even if we don't ride our bike for years our brain will remember how to ride a bike.

Neuroplasticity also means that the brain can learn and adapt in negative ways. This is the case with chronic pain. In this instance, pathways can be sensitized and become more efficient and proficient in signaling the message of pain. The more constant and persistent the signal is along the highway, the more entrenched the signal of pain becomes. Emotions linked to pain can become reinforced as well. At some point along the pathways, changes can even become consistent, and an otherwise short-term, acute pain event can become an entrenched chronic pain problem.

From Acute to Chronic Pain

According to the American Chronic Pain Association, acute pain is *"pain of recent onset, transient, and usually from an identifiable cause."*[4] For instance, a person experiences acute pain following a sprained ankle while playing soccer or after cutting a finger while chopping vegetables.

Many times, acute pain is a symptom of the body's response that contribute to the healing process. These include inflammation, muscle spasm, and even an automatic response, known as fight or flight response. While these are short-lived and natural responses designed to restore the body to its baseline and normal functioning, sometimes they can cause mild or even severe pain, which may be momentary or last several weeks. Acute pain is typically self-limited; once the pain stimulus is resolved or healed, the pain stops.

Chronic pain is pain that lasts even after the injury has otherwise healed. The pain functions more like a disease than a symptom. The pain pathway and its modulators have changed. The pain signal continues to be triggered due to a persistent cause and stimulus.[5]

Over the course of three to six months, if recovery does not occur or if pain is not effectively treated, the body can develop a maladaptive response that can perpetuate and even exacerbate the problem anywhere, and even at multiple points, along the pathway.[6] In other words, the mechanisms in the central nervous system that turn down the volume on pain no longer function properly.

The injury that caused pain may no longer exist, and may have even healed, but the pathway that originally sent the pain message to the brain remains open and unopposed. The brain receives the message of pain even after the original stimulus no longer exists. When this happens, even ordinary touch and pressure can become a source of pain.

Why sensitization happens to some people and not to others is not exactly known. Genetic and environmental factors related to stress may be involved. However, the sensitization develops it is a major player in chronic pain.

What I have experienced and seen: for some people with CRPS it seems like the perfect storm in the brain and body. Many times, there is a drop in the immune system, an incident (injury, accident or surgery), and involvement of stress. This creates a condition where the brain remains open and unopposed. The brain receives the message of pain even after the original stimulus no longer exists and perpetuates chronic pain. When chronic pain continues, it eventually rewires the central nervous system and can cause changes in the brain and spinal cord.

Many of the reflexes that the body has to respond to pain can also be altered. The flight or flight response and other automatic responses may become altered or muted, and coping hormones such as serotonin and other endorphins may become depleted, thus creating a decreased tolerance to pain.[7] If the fight or flight response persists in response to pain, the body can continue to release chemicals that cause muscle spasms and vessel constriction. This limits blood flow and oxygen delivery to the tissues where they are required for healing. This can perpetuate pain in the site. Further, the heart may continue to beat faster, and the person may respond with increased blood pressure. This can lead to an increased consumption of oxygen that would otherwise be used for normal, baseline bodily functions. The body needs to compensate. In an otherwise healthy person, this compensation may be noticeable as decreased energy or fatigue. A person who already has cardiovascular issues may not be able to compensate and their health may become further compromised in response to persistent pain.

A persistent fight or flight response to acute pain may cause a person to develop and maintain a protective posture and to have shallow breathing. This is called splinting, an involuntary response in which a person tightens up to limit movement that causes pain. Over time, the rib cage can develop limited movement, and the abdominal dia-phragm, the muscle that needs to fully move up and down beneath the rib cage to generate airflow in the lungs, becomes tight and restricted. As a result, the person isn't getting oxygen deeply within their tissues when they take a breath. So, there is a marginal deficit in oxygen delivery in the face of increased oxygen demand caused by pain. Another compensation occurs. The body runs on oxygen, and the body needs to compensate for decreased oxygen delivery with energy that would otherwise go towards normal biological functions. This might include corrective measures that would lead to the body normally healing the injury. In an otherwise health person, this compensation might be marginally noticeable as fatigue, but for a person who already has breathing difficulties due to asthma or COPD, this decreased capacity could lead to more respiratory episodes.

Normalizing the Pain Pathways

Changing your brain and your response to pain are key. The brain can modulate or affect pain by directing activity in the nerves and systems beneath it. While some changes within the pain pathway can be permanent, many changes can be reversed or corrected. If the nervous system can change for the negative, it can also change for the positive. This is great news.

So, for effective treatment, it isn't usually just

one pill, one injection, one routine or one exercise that brings about change for healing. Effective treatment involves accessing as many points along the pain pathway as possible and normalizing the message. This is a multimodality approach and is what eventually helped me to gain long-term remission and regain my life.

We have to work with the body as a whole. Neuroplasticity plays a huge part in unraveling chronic pain and helping patients regain function. Add neuroplasticity into a multimodality protocol or program and it can be life changing.

CHAPTER 9

Treatment

One week later I returned to Dr. Amir's office with a family member. We were going to attempt a local or regional block, and we were going to finish a discussion on different types of medications for CRPS. I was apprehensive about another needle being stuck into my foot especially with it as sensitive as it was.

Waiting for my doctor to come into the room was quite the time. There were many obscure comments followed by silence between myself and my family. I could tell that I was not the only one nervous. None of us knew what to expect.

Finally, the tap on the door and in came Dr. Amir. I introduced him to my family member and we got down to business. He started answering questions regarding CRPS, my specific case, there were jokes made about my continually moving little toe, and then he was ready to do the block. The one thing I will say is that Dr. Amir was always caring and compassionate with me. He knew that this would be extremely painful and he took the time to talk me through it.

The first injection of Marcaine and a small amount of cortisone did nothing. I take that back. My fifth toe aka little toe started moving quicker and it hurt like hell. While we were waiting a few minutes to see if there was a delayed response there were many jokes make between my doctor and myself about putting puppets on my toes and making a video. I guess anything to break the tension.

Dr. Amir couldn't understand why the block didn't work. So, he wanted to inject a different area to create a block. Heart pounding, stress levels increasing, face going flush... I just didn't know if I could do this. I told myself I had to try it. I had to give him one more opportunity if I was going to get better.

The second injection into a slightly different area was just as painful and again no block. I started thinking back to when Dr. Hauser tried to inject my foot and was unsuccessful. I talked to Dr. Amir about it and he just shook his head. It just wasn't making sense, but he was not going to continue to poke me for no reason.

Over the span of the next four years it was evident

that the initial estimate of getting into remission in six months to a year was incorrect. During this time I trialed countless medications and if they didn't work they were discontinued. The medications that seemed to help take the edge off the pain or helped me to sleep were continued. Yet as time progressed it took more and more medication to keep up with the progress of the CRPS and the pain.

During this four-year span I returned to physical therapy countless times, worked on desensitization training, had a TENS unit, and did as much research as I could on possible treatment options.

Every follow-up visit came with a caveat of me bringing in information on possible treatment options. Dr. Amir was good at hearing me out, discussing them and if he felt it was worthwhile, he would investigate them.

One visit was filled with a conversation about HBOT (Hyperbaric Oxygen Therapy) for CRPS. There was a doctor on the East Coast touting that he was able to get CRPS patients into remission using HBOT. I followed his write-ups and researched his website. Armed with information and the fact that I could do HBOT locally I wanted Dr. Amir's input. He was willing to go along with it, but he was not convinced it would work. It would require a prescription from him for me to have access to HBOT at a local clinic and he was willing to write it. He stressed that insurance would not pay for this treatment but if it could help I really didn't care.

I pursued HBOT at a local wellness clinic. I went three times a week for nine or ten weeks. The sessions started off at a lower pressure level and it was gradually increased. I had scuba dived prior to this, so the pressure did not bother me. Week after week I kept expecting to see a big difference in my pain levels but it just didn't happen. I didn't know if it was due to my CRPS being surgically induced or if we were missing something. During my sessions not only did I reach out to the clinic on the East Coast but so did Dr. Amir. We both wanted to know if something else needed to be added to their protocol that he had been given. We were told, no. So, one more protocol down and one more flop.

I started a series of Lumbar Sympathetic Blocks since nothing else seemed to be working. I did my homework on what was involved, risks vs benefits, and any other information I could find.

All of my blocks were done at an outpatient surgery center. The first one I was extremely nervous. After the initial paperwork, signing in and waiting; I was finally called back. I kept telling myself to calm down, but I could feel the anxiety creeping up. I changed into my hospital gown and returned to my gurney. Part of my procedure as with many is the starting of the IV. Easier said than done. My veins are awful. It took three nurses multiple attempts and finally they asked the anesthesiologist to start the IV. Then the next fun part. Getting a temperature reading on my left foot (affected foot) and then my right foot. I had to laugh because the nurses couldn't get a temperature on my left foot because it was so cold. Dr. Amir came in and explained how CRPS worked and told them following the Lumbar Sympathetic Block it would warm up. I was making quite the impression.

Versed was pushed via IV, but as usual it didn't make a difference. Then I was wheeled back to the OR. I helped position myself on the OR table and then they were supposed to do a 'twilight' sedation. They don't want you to feel pain, but they need you to be able to respond to commands. One slight problem I was on so many opioid medications by this point that the Versed and Fentanyl mix that they normally use was just not working. I would start to go out to la-la land and then in a matter of minutes it was wearing off. I could feel everything that was happening, not just pressure, but pain. I was fully aware of the complete conversations in the OR. I tried to move a little to get their attention but it didn't seem to work. I was there face down with tears rolling from my eyes as I told myself that this had to be over soon and I kept reassuring myself that I could do it.

In the PACU area Dr. Amir came by to check on me. My body temperature was extremely low so they were trying to warm me up. My body was in shock from what I had just been through. I still had tears flowing when Dr. Amir tried to assure me that everything was ok. I told him it wasn't. I started to tell him what I felt, what happened and why I was crying. At first he said it was impossible with the medication he had given me, but then he paused. He was beside himself and said it wouldn't happen again.

I met with Dr. Amir in his office as a follow-up and to talk about the Lumbar Sympathetic Block (LSB). He wanted to do a series of them because he felt the block was successful. Yet after my experience I wanted nothing more to do with any blocks. He assured me that it would never happen again. He would personally take control over the medication and if needed we would pull in an anesthesiologist to do a general.

The one thing that we both could put our finger on with regard to what happened was the pure amount of opioid medications that I was on and had been on for several years. Your body builds up a tolerance. This tends to be a problem when patients need a sedation because it is acting on the same receptor sites.

Two weeks later I returned to the outpatient surgery center for my second LSB. Revisiting the previous LSB in my mind made my anticipation and anxiety grow with every passing minute. I knew that I was told this would be different, but how could I be sure.

Here we go. My name was called and the dance began. Grab the hospital gown, empty the bladder, return to the gurney and wait to be used as a pin cushion. The nurses remembered me. Imagine that. They started with a warm pack on my arm and brought out the nursing supervisor to start the IV this time. It only took her two attempts before getting the IV started. Dr. Amir was quick to stop by once he arrived to reassure me that he would be in charge of the medications in the OR and he would make sure everything was ok. He promised.

They started with increasing the Versed given via IV prior to going to the OR. Unfortunately, that did nothing. I enjoyed my ride back to the OR and a quick chat on the way. Once again I helped to position myself on the OR table and then the fun began. Dr. Amir had them push twice the amount of medication as in the previous procedure. He then waited a few minutes and I heard him telling the nursing staff and x-ray tech what was happening. He asked how I was and I was still having a complete conversation with him. He instructed the nurse to push additional medication and then started the LSB. He had one of the nurses checking on me and I could tell he was concerned. Just a few minutes in the exact same thing happened. I came out of sedation, felt a sharp pain and started to move. He must have been at a critical spot in the block because he told me not to move as he completely stopped what he was doing and raised his voice. The nurse didn't want to push any additional medication and Dr. Amir yelled back that he was instructing them to do it. It was a big ta-do in the OR. He eventually finished the block but it was not a good situation for anyone.

In the PACU he once again came to check on me. I was frustrated and was trying not to cry but I couldn't help it. I just couldn't do this. I couldn't be tortured in hope that it would help my CRPS. It was agreed that we would finish discussing it in his office.

Following the first two blocks it was decided that any further LSB would have to be done with a general anesthesia. That was the only safe way to do it with me, so that is how we proceeded.

There were a total of eleven more LSB completed. Following each block my affected foot and ankle would increase in temperature, but it didn't give me a lot of pain relief. Yet, they were considered a success.

After lucky number thirteen I started to swell up.

I had a really puffy face, I just felt out of sorts, I was extremely tired and didn't feel well. I had a follow-up visit with my Neurologist and she immediately noticed the difference in my appearance. She was wanting to know what was happening, symptoms and any procedures that I may have done. We talked about the Lumbar Sympathetic Blocks. She was concerned about possible adrenal issues and sent me directly to the ER.

Within a matter of minutes I was at the ER and being seen. Blood was drawn, urine samples, etc. All I knew was I was in pain, but worst of all I just felt like crap. It didn't take very long for the doctor to come in to discuss my test results and start asking if I had ever had any adrenal or kidney issues. No. Why all the questions about adrenals? Well, apparently I was in adrenal failure.

The paperwork was started and I was told that I was being admitted. Just what I didn't want to hear.

Taking a ride up to my assigned room in a hospital bed. The sights, sounds and smells of a hospital are just difficult to block out. It was not a place that I wanted to be and not anything that I was looking forward to. I was still in shock that I was being told that I was in adrenal failure. How could this happen after a series of Lumbar Sympathetic

Blocks? Now what? I had no answers.

My pain management doctor and Neurologist were notified of my admission and they were both on staff at the hospital. I was assigned an Endocrinologist from the on call staff. One school of thought was to just give it time and to keep me for observation. The other thought was to start me on medication to try to jump start my adrenal glands. It was the second group that won out.

How anyone can become accustomed to a hospital is beyond me. The constant prodding, stats, blood draws, beeping and noise around you is overwhelming. The first day was manageable as I was in the room by myself. Then things changed as I received an older roommate that was quite the handful. Add in moaning, groaning, yelling for the nurse and a constant ruckus and now I was more than ready to be discharged as soon as humanly possible.

After three days of little sleep and many distractions something was beginning to work. My adrenal function was increasing. This was fantastic news as there was talk about me going home. Hallelujah.

Once released I found a new Endocrinologist that I was comfortable with, and he put me on a supplement to increase adrenal function rather than putting me on prescription medications. This made me very happy and it was working. After a couple of months new bloodwork was completed and we found that my adrenal function was back to normal.

Follow-up visits with Dr. Amir continued through this time too. We discussed what happened and although it was rare it was a possible side effect of doing too many blocks too close together and having a reaction to the Cortisone. This is what happened to me.

CHAPTER 10

Stress and Pain

Things hurt more when we are stressed, sad or anxious, and the increased pain makes us feel stressed, sad and anxious. The way out of this vicious cycle is a whole change to how we perceive fear, suffering and setbacks.

"I'm stressed out, tired, exhausted and in pain." These are words that are all to common to CRPS and chronic pain patients. The words reflect a growing state of people in all walks of life that are affected by chronic pain. If you feel overwhelmed by the demands of family, work, school, etc., you are not alone.

Stress is a product of our postmodern life. We feel we have to little time, too few resources, and a lack of control over most things in our lives. Stress can be related to life transitions, the environment, individual growth, a desire for healing, lack of understanding, or a perception of things. Stress can be generated by an event such as an illness, a diagnosis, or a bad decision. Some stressful events, like the birth of a baby, are positive and predictable. Others, such as a natural disaster and an injury, are not. When stress is negative and unpredictable, it can be hard to manage.

How we react to stress is the key to keeping it in check. If we carry stress in our bodies and minds, it disrupts our sense of wellbeing. Thus, it interferes with the mental and physical rest we need. Unmanaged stress can lead to the development of anxiety disorders, depression, and physical symptoms, including pain.

Stress is a part of life. There is good stress and bad stress. Stress can be a good motivator, but too much of it or ongoing stress can be problematic. When stress is present, the brain releases chemicals and hormones; heart rate and blood pressure increase; and the immune system is activated. You become tense and constricted in your muscles, which lead you to feel tired. Chronic stress causes repeat surges of cortisol, resulting in cortisol dysfunction and inflammation.[8] Then muscles tense up making the pain worse. Your brain has trouble filtering your pain signals. Over time, you stressed brain gets more and more sensitized to processing pain and it takes less and less stimuli to experience it.[9] The body wants balance. Pain and stress disrupt this. The body attempts to adapt to stress and pain, but after a while, it is challenged by both. Pain and stress create constant wear and tear on the body and emotions.

Another reason why stress affects pain is due to the fact that the stress response also affects the limbic system in the brain. The prefrontal region of the brain and limbic system (ACC, amygdala, VTA, and NAc) are associated with affective aspects of pain and regulate emotional and motivational responses. These brain regions are not activated separately; they are functionally connected and contribute in a combined fashion to pain processing. Changes in emotional and motivational cues can affect the intensity and degree of pain experience. [10] Therefore, when our stress increases our pain increases.

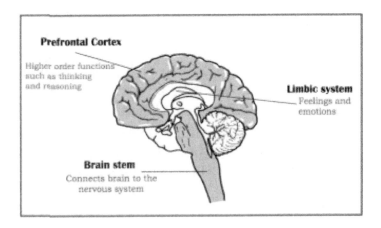

Prefrontal Cortex
Higher order functions
such as thinking
and reasoning

Limbic system
Feelings and
emotions

Brain stem
Connects brain to the
nervous system

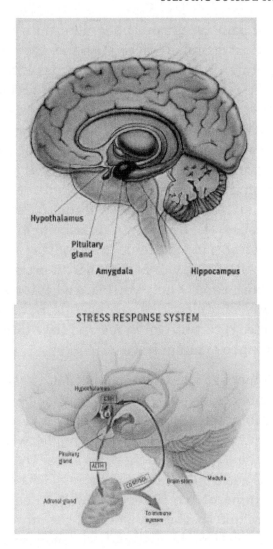

The Brain's Role

The brain plays a role in processing of stress and

chronic pain. When our body determines a situation is stressful, it activates the part of the autonomic nervous system that goes into fight or flight response. This triggers the activation of our central stress response system called the hypothalamic-pituitary-adrenal (HPA) axis and leads to a release of adrenal glucocorticoids. [11] These hormones have receptors in the emotional processing center of the brain called the limbic system and impact cell functioning.[12] Perceived stress causes the limbic system to remember and pay attention and to decide to flee or stay in a situation. All of this works together to protect you from danger and to help you learn what is not safe. Basically, chronic stress causes your nervous system to go into survival mode and have difficulty returning to a calmer state.

Researchers at the University of Montreal studied the relationship between stress and pain from a neurobiological standpoint. They conducted a pain study and found a relationship between the size of the structures in the brain called the hippocampus and a vulnerability to stress. The smaller the volume of the hippocampus (the center of memory and spatial navigation), the more stress (higher cortisol levels) and, consequently, the more pain. [13] And there was more activity in the part of the brain (anterior parahippocampal gyrus) related to anxiety over anticipation of pain.

Response to Stress

Reducing life stress will improve the quality of our lives. Why? Physically, stress drains us. Psychologically, stress affects our ability to think clearly, remember things, make good decisions and regulate your emotions. Most importantly, eliminating stress can physically alter our vulnerability to recurring pain.

Stress of all types can make pain worse if it's not managed or controlled. A key component of living beyond pain is to manage stress and develop good coping skills. We are capable of modifying what we perceive as stressful and of responding to stress in adaptive ways. Also, the more we can eliminate or avoid stress triggers, the better our stress management will be. Stress affects our pain and dials it up if not well managed.

For me the stress of even thinking about a spinal cord stimulator was causing added stress. I was quickly finding out how big the stress response played into increasing my pain.

CHAPTER 11

Spinal Cord Stimulators

After a couple of months passed of numerous appointments with Dr. Amir and added medications, I was not progressing. As a matter of fact my pain, swelling and coloration changes were getting worse. The frustration was real. I was realizing very quickly that this was more than just the pain, it was more than just an inconvenience. It was something that was affecting my entire body, my outlook, how I responded to those around me and so much more.

Dr. Amir thought it was time for a more drastic approach. He revisited the idea of a Spinal Cord Stimulator (SCS). Of course the first thing out of my mouth was, "*NO*." I had a hard time wrapping my head around something foreign in my body and could not see how a SCS could possibly stop my CRPS. Dr. Amir took the time to describe the trial and the procedure with the help of a poster that was conveniently located in each treatment room. The goal is to have the leads or paddle on specific nerves. When turned on the SCS would then send a different signal to the brain other than pain.

Very thin wires called leads were responsible for delivering the electrical impulses to the nerves along the specific area on the spine. Other times they utilize a paddle - which allows them to cover a larger area. They then connect a battery in the upper buttocks area or hip. The battery produces the intensity of the electrical current or signal sent through the leads or paddle, which are programed and controlled through a remote control.

Prior to having the real deal implanted every patient goes through a trial with a SCS. This could be three days or it could be a week. It all depends on their doctor and diagnosis. Dr. Amir explained that a trial SCS would be placed so the leads were implanted and then the wires were on the outside of the body. The battery would be worn around the waist in something like a fanny pack. Oh, don't forget the remote to control the stimulation.

There was a lot of information given in a very short period of time. It was a lot to digest. I needed time to think about this and to talk with my family. This was a big deal, and I needed time to make the best decision possible. Dr. Amir sent me home with a folder that included information and a DVD to watch.

I started reading the information shortly after arriving home but I just couldn't bring myself to watch the DVD. I discussed my visit with the doctor and sat down together with my family to watch the DVD. It presented the basic facts and made it sound like the glorious answer, but something in my gut just kept gnawing at me. Of course the decision was left for me to make knowing I would have full support regardless of what I decided.

I did more research online and jumped onto the online support groups to see if anyone else had any experience with a SCS. I heard bits and pieces but nothing that was convincing me one way or the other. This had to be a personal decision based on where I was at the time.

Wanting more time to mull it over, I waited several days prior to making the call. I was ready to move forward with the trial of the SCS. Dr. Amir was more than pleased with my decision. I was scheduled in the following week for the trial.

Counting down the days, each day that got closer was filled with anxiety. I kept wondering if I made the right decisions. My mind was playing tricks with me. I wanted so badly for something to work at this point, but I was jaded because nothing had.

This is the point where you feel that you've lost

control. The loss is palpable. The want and need to regain that control is immense.

I remember sitting at the surgery center wondering what the heck I was doing. What had I gotten myself into? Then I heard my name called and there was no more time for speculation. It was game time. As a frequent flier - of surgeries and procedures - I knew the drill all too well. Basic questions, change into hospital gown, empty bladder, return to assigned gurney, more vital signs, start IV and then the real fun begins.

After getting settled I had a Medtronic representative come in to meet me. I guess it didn't dawn on me that she would be at my surgery much less in the OR. She was going over the specifics of the trial SCS, what would happen in the procedure/surgery and that they would need me awake during portions of it so they would know for sure if the leads were placed correctly. STOP right there! Awake during portions? This would mean trying to use a twilight sedation and from my past experiences with that I knew all too well that was not going to work. Panic set in and she could tell. I'm not sure that she could put her finger on exactly what caused the increase in blood pressure, the flushed look on my face or the exasperation – but she knew something she said did it. I think that was probably the quickest she had left the bedside to try to get a nurse or doctor.

Dr. Amir returned with the Medtronic representative and wanted to know what my concerns
were. I explained that there was no way that we
were going to move forward with this if it was
planned with a twilight sedation. As I started to
remind him of the Lumbar Sympathetic Blocks he
stopped me. He acknowledged the issues I had
with sedation and assured me that this would be
done with a general anesthetic. It was unusual
to do it this way, but in my case it was the only
safe way to proceed. Those were the words that I
needed to hear.

A few minutes later I was wheeled back to the OR,
where I was positioned face down on my stomach.
The OR is extremely cold and being face down is
not the most comfortable position. I was thankful the anesthesiologist was there and that it was
going to be a general. In a matter of minutes the
room faded to black and I was in my own world.

I awoke in the PACU. There was more information
to learn prior to being discharged about restric-
tions, how to work the SCS, not showering, etc.
I had a follow-up appointment set the following
day to meet with Dr. Amir and the Medtronic rep
to make sure everything was ok.

That night was not the most pleasant. I was still

groggy from the anesthesia but my back was sore from the procedure and I still had pain in my foot and ankle. I was unable to lay on my back instead I had to figure out how to comfortably sleep on my side propped up with pillows.

The next day I met with my doctor and the Medtronic rep was there. She spent more time with me then my doctor did, so I guess this appointment was more about meeting with her than anything. She made adjustments to the frequencies and intensity, plugged in settings and set up the remote so that I was getting some relief.

I left the office that day determined to find out if the SCS really worked. I wanted to put it to the test one way or the other. So, over the next few days I walked in grass barefoot, walked in sand barefoot, put my affected foot in a swimming pool that was not exactly warm and did multiple other things that in the past would have set off my CRPS. This time with the SCS trial I was managing to get through these things. I was intrigued. Perhaps this could be the answer.

One week later I returned to my doctor's office to have the leads removed and to discuss moving forward with the real SCS. I saw the results of the trial which were nothing but fascinating, but my gut was still in knots over this decision.

Dr. Amir referred me over to a top Neurosurgeon to have the actual SCS placed. He felt this was the best way of moving forward. So, over the next couple of weeks I had to meet with Dr. Holmes; a neurosurgeon; to see if he felt I was a proper candidate. This seemed a little antiquated since I just did a SCS trial, but I knew that I had to play by the rules.

My first appointment with Dr. Holmes went well. His lobby was filled to capacity with patients and he was running behind, but I guess this is normal. When I was finally called back he gave me 100% of his attention. He had already reviewed my medical records and was very thorough. Although the trial was considered a success he still wanted a full brain and spine CT prior to moving forward. He went over the way he did the implant of a SCS and answered all of the questions that were posed that day.

I returned for my second appointment to receive the results of the CT and to see where things stood. On one hand he said, "*You have a perfect spine which I normally don't see... this makes me not want to do a surgery on you.*" He knew that any implantation could and most likely would change the spine. He also knew the pain that I was living with. Both Dr. Amir and Dr. Holmes agreed that the SCS was my best option at this time. I discussed my concerns with him regarding possible sedation vs a

general anesthetic. He said based upon my medication list they would use a general and he would
also keep me in-patient due to concerns over pain
control. I talked with him at length about the
possibility of the implant surgery of the spinal
cord stimulator causing my CRPS to move into
my back. I was told this had never happened and
there was not literature to back up this concern.
After going over any further questions the surgery
was scheduled.

The day of reckoning came. It was the big day
for the implantation of the real SCS. The biggest
thought going through my head was, "... *what the
heck am I doing?*" This was followed by the hope
and many prayers that this would actually allow
me to regain my life.

I had done my research prior to this and I knew
that a SCS would not stop the possible progression
of the CRPS, but is could dramatically decrease my
pain levels. This was the goal.

I knew the routine all too well. I had had too many
procedures and surgeries to date. I arrived at the
hospital with my family and we were nervous.
We had trust in Dr. Holmes, but with everything I
had been through we all knew that no surgery was
going to be easy.

The waiting was always the worst part. Sitting

in the cold, sterile, uninviting waiting room to be called back. Not knowing what to say. Butterflies in my stomach. Anxiety increasing with every tick of the clock. Then you hear your name and the time has come.

Different place, different time, but the routine was all too well known. Proper identification of patient, assigned gurney, grab a lovely surgical gown (opening in the back), empty bladder, and return to gurney to start IV. It is pathetic when the patient can anticipate what is going to happen prior to the nurses asking.

I saw the Medtronic rep roaming around the nursing station and then she disappeared. She finally came into talk with me and started to explain the procedure to me. I stopped her in her tracks when she started to tell me that they bring the patients out of anesthesia to test the SCS to ensure proper placement. This was not on my radar and it was just not going to happen. My experience with sedation, the amount of medications I was on, and the inability to keep me sedated was just not an option. The panic button was hit. The look on my face, the increase in my blood pressure, the red blotchy coloration that happens when I am anxious – it was all happening. I was on the verge of calling off the entire surgery when Dr. Holmes walked in with the anesthesiologist. There was no waiting for the, *"Do you have any questions?"*

There were a ton of concerns flowing out of my mouth at a million miles a minute. To the point that Dr. Holmes finally stopped me with his calm demeanor and reiterated that this would not be the routine SCS surgery. He was fully aware of my medications, past history and he had spoken with the anesthesiologist to ensure that a general would be used through the entire procedure. There would be no need to test the SCS as he knew exactly where it needed to be placed. He also impressed and reiterated that I would be kept in ICU to control my pain for at least the first 24 hours.

I felt better hearing all of this but I still had a big concern weighing heavily on my mind so I asked. *"Do we need to take any additional precautions to make sure my CRPS doesn't spread with this surgery?"* I was told we had already discussed this and it never happens. There was nothing to be worried about. It would be fine.

Dr. Holmes left my bedside to get prepped for the surgery while the anesthesiologist pushed Versed into my IV. I laughed as he was trying to describe to me that I may feel a little sleepy. I told him that Versed never works due to the amount of meds that I took on a daily basis. It was quite an interesting back and forth as he just stood there waiting for it to take affect all the while I just continued the conversation. He left the area with additional orders of Versed to be pushed again prior to heading back to the OR.

The time had come to head back. The additional Versed was administered into my IV, the goodbyes were said and off we went. The corridors to the OR were always filled with various equipment and carts. As soon as you enter into the OR it is distinctively cold and sterile with a specific smell. All with a hustle and bustle of those trying to make sure everything is in its exact place. This is when you know there is no turning back. The stress and anxiety levels are increasing, stomach is churning and you just wonder what the heck you are doing – all simultaneously while being instructed and helped over to a narrow, cold OR table. Nurses and the anesthesiologist all trying to get things in place. Because this was a Spinal Cord Stimulator I had to be face down (not the most comfortable) blood pressure cuff on, pulse ox on, arm out on side extension for easy access to IV and monitoring, etc. Once the medication started to flow into the IV I could feel a warmth in my body and then the familiar fuzzy feeling before going out.

I awoke in PACU for a short while and was immediately transferred to the ICU. At first everything was just a blur. That night I remember the nurses being extremely attentive and making sure that my pain levels were under control. It was definitely not a night of sleep. It was more like drifting in and out due to all of the pain medications free flowing as they were trying to keep me comfortable until the next morning when they were going to turn on the SCS.

Morning arrived and I heard a knock at the door and a familiar face of the Medtronic representative as she introduced herself again as she walked into the room. It was her job to show me how to properly use the SCS; actually the remote; and to care for the device. We had already spoken about a lot of this, but it was important to go over all the details more in-depth. She would need to program in different programs into the remote based upon many different things such as area of stimulation, intensity and frequency. The time came to turn on the SCS to see where the stimulation was reaching and what was needed to program different settings on the remote. At first it felt like I had a little alien in my body as I was trying to concentrate on exactly where I was feeling any sensations. I had so much medication flowing through me that it was difficult to concentrate and to differentiate the stimulation from my pain. Eventually we were able to set up several programs to help cover my left foot and ankle, left leg and my right leg (as there were times the CRPS was trying to mirror).

A bit later Dr. Holmes came in and wanted to know how the SCS was doing. We talked about the incisional pain in my back and hip due to the surgery in comparison to the CRPS pain. He was going to have me moved from ICU to a regular room to make sure I could control my pain with medication and the SCS prior to being released. We were all in agreement on this.

Finally being back home was a relief in and of itself. My back was still painful from undergoing a spinal procedure. It was nearly impossible to find a comfortable position. Before it was only my foot and ankle that I needed to worry about, but now it was also my back and hip. I knew pillows would be my friend in the coming days.

The spinal cord stimulator in and of itself was quite the thing. Every time I would turn it on or change the settings I felt like I had an alien inside of me. It is just so hard to describe. It was a constant buzzing feeling; they call it stimulation; that was difficult to adjust to. When I would turn down the stimulator due to the annoyance then it didn't cover my pain as well. If I turned it up to high then I felt like it was taking over my body. I was overwhelmed trying to find that setting that was just right.

I was pushing myself to take little walks at the park. To get out of the house a bit more and to try to see how this new SCS was really going to help me compared to the trial. Thus far I was not impressed.

I made an appointment to meet with my Medtronic rep to adjust the stimulation and frequencies. I was told it was just a matter of fine tuning it so that it would work better for me and then I would be on the road to recovery. I felt like a robot getting reprogrammed during that time. Having her look at a computer screen making adjustments and having to report what I was feeling and where I was feeling it. Was it a buzzing, a sharp or dull pain, was it too high or too low, etc. I was essentially being reprogrammed. Wow! This was not exactly what I had signed up for and I was not too comfortable going through this for close to an hour. We were finally able to zero in on several programs that were better than where I was previously. Now it was time to see how they worked.

I had been utilizing my SCS off and on for a couple weeks and it was time to charge it. I was anxious about doing this but everyone kept telling me it wasn't a big deal. It is just an external device that you wear over the battery for approximately 45 minutes to an hour to charge it. I finally figured out the placement and laid propped up on pillows while it was charging. I noticed during this time that my foot was throbbing a bit but didn't think too much about it. 50 minutes later I was done charging the battery, my foot felt like it was on fire and when I looked it was swollen up 2-3 times its normal size. Oh my gosh, what this normal? Had I done something wrong?

I contacted my pain management doctor to find out what I was supposed to do. I was a little panicked to say the least. He was not convinced it had anything to do with the battery charging as he had never heard of anything like this, but told me to elevate my foot and increase my NSAIDS. I already had a follow-up appointment the following week so we left that alone. My mind was racing, foot was pounding and burning, and I just couldn't wrap my head around all of this. Feeling defeated I headed to bed hoping for the best.

The next day, I was still not feeling better. The pain continued in my foot and ankle, and the swelling was persistent. Yes, it had gone down a little but it had not resolved. Somewhat afraid to turn on the spinal cord stimulator I knew I had to do something to try to calm down the pain. Yes, I still had all of my pain medication and I was still taking it. There just had to be a better way.

Reluctant I grabbed my remote and turned on the stimulator. I knew I had to give it a good college try. I was still having problems getting use to the weird tingling and buzzing feeling every time I used it.

This unusual response to the charging of the battery mystified my doctors in addition to the

Medtronic representative. Everyone wanted to dismiss it and say it was a fluke, but I was just not convinced.

My incisions were checked thoroughly and were healing perfectly. Nothing had shifted at the battery site and everyone kept reiterating that nothing was out of place and I was healing well.

The settings were checked on the stimulator, some adjustments were made and I was told to have some patience. No one wanted to make any rash decisions and they were convinced this was the Holy Grail to solve the chronic pain/CRPS pain. I only wish that I was that convinced.

I had learned to listen to my body and know when something was wrong, but I had to be able to show them I was right.

Over the next few weeks I continued to use the stimulator as directed, and every time I would charge the batter the same thing would happen. My left foot would swell up like a balloon. I finally got smart and took pictures of it so that I could send them to my doctor(s). Once they saw the same thing that I was living with the decision was made that a rechargeable battery was not an option for me.

Neither my pain management doctor nor Dr. Holmes; my neurosurgeon; wanted to completely remove the spinal cord stimulator. They were both still convinced that it would help reduce my pain and give me a better quality of life if they could resolve the battery issue. I on the other hand was not convinced. I was willing to go along because I had to find something that would help me – I was desperate.

There were many meetings, conversations and conference calls between Medtronic, my doctors and me. No one could explain why charging a battery could possibly cause the reaction of swelling in an affected limb. Regardless, it was decided that removing the rechargeable battery and replacing it with a non-rechargeable battery would be the best solution. Until this could be done I turned off the stimulator since it was causing more problems and pain than it was resolving.

Dr. Holmes had me get a full set of X-Rays of my spine to verify the placement of the paddle and to ensure that nothing had moved prior to the surgery. Everything looked good. He said the placement was perfect, nothing had shifted and it was a green light to just replace the battery.

Following the surgery to change out the battery I had many appointment to manipulate the stimulator's frequency and to set up new programs. Something was just off. It seemed like every week I had to make a call into my pain management doctor to complain about the stimulator. It got to the point that I was assigned a Regional Manager from Medtronic that would meet me to trouble shoot my system.

My incisions had completely healed up but my back was still having some pain that was not there prior to the surgery. It was difficult for me to pinpoint what was going on but I knew it was not quite right.

The weeks turned into months and I continued to have even more issues with the stimulator. Depending on the setting and program I would have a weird shocking sensation. I was having problems getting the same coverage that I had in the beginning. There were a couple times when I had the stimulator on coming down my stairs that it went haywire, I couldn't feel my foot and ended up falling. This was just not a good combination for someone dealing with CRPS. It was not taking away my pain, I was not dealing with even more issues and I was getting overwhelmed.

I met with Dr. Holmes again and he could not figure out why I would be having any problem with the stimulator as the only change was the battery. He had new X-Rays taken and there was no change in the placement of the paddle. There had to be an issue with the stimulator.

On the other side Medtronic did not want to be held responsible for any malfunction and kept wanting to blame Dr. Holmes. They kept stating that the paddle must have shifted or it was not placed correctly if this was happening. Essentially I was caught in the middle.

I was doing everything I could do as a patient to advocate for myself. I was speaking with my pain management doctor; Dr. Amir; working with Dr. Holmes and working with Medtronic. I was going above and beyond. I even did an online search to see if there were any FDA reports about this issue. I felt like I had been dropped into the pit of hell.

To be honest, I didn't care who did what or if no one was to blame. I was not playing a blame game. All I wanted was some answer and a resolve so that I could move forward in regaining my life. Getting stuck between a top neurosurgeon and a DME company is not my idea of fun.

I was tired and just wanted it removed. Dr. Amir on the other hand didn't want to remove it without having something to replace it because he was running out of solutions. He brought in a top representative from Boston Scientific and had me meet with him. We went over all the issues I had been dealing with since day one. I explained all of my concerns and laid out on the table that I was very hesitant about moving forward with another stimulator. I wanted to know what made their system different and why I should consider it. He did his best to assure me that Boston Scientific would make their top representative available to me and discussed the advantages of their stimulator. I was still not convinced but was sent home with their information and DVD to watch.

That night I sat with my family to go over the information, talk about concerns and to brainstorm. I was overwhelmed. My gut told me to just have the stimulator removed and move on to something else, but I had an immense amount of pressure on me. I was told there was nothing else. I had to think of my family – my son.

If this is the **only** thing that my doctors have to offer and I am running out of FDA approved treatment options – then I guess I have to try it again. My heart was heavy and my stomach was churning as I made this decision to move forward.

Once again I found myself in the all too familiar hospital waiting room waiting to be called back for another surgery. This was huge. Ultimately, it was my decision, but my brain and my gut were in a tug-of-war over the decision that was made. I sat there in silence. Time slowly clicked by on the clock as I wondered when I would be called back so that I could just get this over with.

Once called back I knew what to do. All I needed to know was what gurney I was assigned to. I knew what information the nurse needed, I understood what would be asked of me and then let the circus begin. It is like the Hokey Pokey. Left arm in; id bracelet; left arm out and shake it all about... right arm in; IV – hopefully; right arm out... you get the drift. When your nerves are on high alert you better find some humor in things.

Once the IV is in place, the paperwork and vital signs are done then family can come back and the doctors will come in. Routine. I met with Dr. Holmes as usual to go over the surgery and ask any further questions. Again, I asked about the possibility of my CRPS advancing into my back. I asked about the possibility of utilizing Ketamine during the surgery and I was told it wasn't needed... "There is nothing to worry about."

I was uneasy with this surgery. Removing a stimulator and replacing it. This seemed like a big deal to me. I always got a little nervous before any surgery but this one had me on edge. It is hard to describe the feeling that you get in the pit of your stomach or the thousands of thoughts that run through your head.

The time had come to be wheeled back, to say my good bye and to move into the cold sterile area known as the OR.

I woke up in the PACU (post-anesthesia care unit)

groggy, in pain and not knowing what was happening. The medication from the surgery had not worn off yet; I was nauseous and trying to reorient. As more pain medication was administered to keep me comfortable I drifted back out. I came to a bit later with my family by my side trying to answer my questions and explain what happened.

Although I appreciated the information there was no way I was going to remember what was said because I was under the influence to too many medications. It was time to be moved from the PACU into a room upstairs. All I knew was that I was uncomfortable, my back hurt and I couldn't focus on anything happening.

I switched beds very gingerly, and the staff reconnected all the machines. The nursing staff was monitoring all my vital signs and pain levels to ensure that everything was going as smoothly as possible.

The following morning I had the Boston Scientific representative knocking on my door and coming to program their stimulator. I guess it was now my stimulator. With the vast amount of medication I was on it was very difficult for me to distinguish the stimulation, different frequencies and answer all of the questions. I did my best, but I was exhausted. We would meet again once I was discharged.

I had high hopes leaving the hospital. I wanted

this stimulator to work in the worst way. I would give anything to get my life back, so this just had to work.

The normal follow up visit with Dr. Holmes was the week following my surgery. My incision was red and itchy. They had used staples on the incision to close the top layer and I was having an allergic reaction. I was also allergic to Steri-Strips so we had limited options on keeping the incision closed while it healed. The staples were removed, a surgical glue was applied with gauze and paper tape to protect the area. From the looks of it things were healing up well.

I had noticed that I was having some neuropathic pain in my back around my incisions. I was afraid to call it CRPS but I did ask Dr. Holmes about it. He had noticed when he removed the staples that I was extra sensitive to touch and was a little concerned. He reiterated that this had never happened with any other patient before. I think we were both thinking the same thing but neither of us wanted to say the words.

Following this appointment I met with the Boston Scientific rep. We needed to make adjustments to the settings and frequencies. It was important to try to hone in as much as possible in the areas that would give me the most relief at the lowest intensity levels. One it was more comfortable and secondly it would allow the battery to last longer.

I also met with Dr. Amir regarding the CRPS in my back. It was hard to fathom how the surgeries to place the stimulators could have caused the CRPS to move. I asked so many times if this was possible and everyone said, NO. Yet here I am living with the pain and it is spreading.

Within the first 90 days I had met with the Boston Scientific rep countless times. Each time we were having to increase the intensity and change the frequencies to try to manage the pain. They were concerned that I would get to the point that the SCS would no longer control the pain because it was unusual to make dramatic increases in such a short span of time. There was something else going on and we needed to pin-point it.

I spoke with Dr. Amir and Dr. Holmes regarding the concerns and at the same time so did Boston Scientific. The concern was there was a layer of scar tissue building up in the area that was prohibiting the signal from getting to the nerves. We needed to figure this out. The big problem we had with the stimulator is once it is placed you can no longer do a MRI. Instead an ultrasound was done in the area and it was confirmed that there was a build-up of scar tissue on the area of the dura.

This presented an even bigger question and an urgent question. Were there any write-ups on scar tissue on the dura secondary to a spinal cord stimulator? If, yes, what were the outcomes and what did we need to do?

Dr. Holmes did a search for any published articles on this subject and sent me back an email with an attachment within 24 hours. The specific article was about a patient that received a spinal cord stimulator for chronic pain, following placement had a build-up of scar tissue on the dura that compressed the spine and lead to paralysis from the waist down. They had to do a spinal decompression and other procedure to allow the patient to regain movement in their legs.

This was all I needed to read to know that I had to get a surgery scheduled ASAP to get this stimulator removed. I was living a horror story and when I thought it couldn't get any worse it did.

Everyone was great with getting the surgery scheduled as quickly as possible, working together as a team to make sure that everything would go smoothly while trying to meet my needs. I signed off on paperwork that would allow Dr. Holmes to write up my case and submit it to be published so that others would know the possible draw backs of spinal cord stimulators. The big question to me is whether other doctors actually took the time to read these published articles or if they only looked them up with cases like mine. I will never know this answer.

Once the spinal cord stimulator was removed it was reiterated that my doctors were out of treatment options. The best they could do was to keep me as comfortable as possible on pain medications. I was floored. This was unacceptable. There had to be another way, another treatment out there that could help, something...

Sitting in the office with Dr. Amir we were talking about my CRPS and how it progressed into my back. He was shaking his head and saying he just didn't have anything else to offer when I insisted that he pull in his partner to discuss this. I insisted there had to be another option out there. I refused to give in and wouldn't leave until Dr. Who came in to consult. Dr. Who had seen me in the hospital and knew exactly what I had been through.

A few minutes later Dr. Who was being pulled from an exam room to discuss the case. He was updated on the last stimulator, the explant and where we were at. I pleaded with both of them to find something - anything that could help me. They talked and went over my file. Finally they both shook their heads and said there was nothing else available. They were sorry, and Dr. Who left the room. Dr. Amir wrote out my prescriptions, gave me a gentle hug and told me he would see me back in a couple weeks.

I was in awe; my whole being was shattered. To hear your doctor, actually 2 doctors say, *"There is nothing else we can do except keep you on medication..."* is numbing. There had to be a way through this. There had to be a way to decrease my pain and regain my life, and I was not going to stop until I figured it out.

Driving home from that appointment I felt like I had been hit over the head with a 2x4. My mind was racing. I was thinking about all the research I had done up to that point and the possible treatments I had looked at: Ketamine Infusions, Ketamine Coma in Mexico; Calmare, etc. Yet, none of these treatment options seemed viable. There were no long-term studies on high dose Ketamine and possible side-effects. Calmare was new and they could not present me with any outcomes. They just said they were sure it would help, but it could take several treatments and require follow up treatments to stay pain free. What about long-term relief? Is it possible? Everyone had an opinion but none that included remission.

There were many, many conversations between myself and family. What do I do, how do I move forward, and what treatment options are even available?

CHAPTER 12

Malpractice

In addition to dealing with everything else I had decided to move forward with a malpractice case against Dr. Hauser. This had nothing to do with money but everything to do with trying to get his license. If he had done this much damage to me and caused this much harm - what had he done to others?

There was a lot of serious consideration that went into filing this case. I found out early on that CRPS is very difficult to prove in a court of law. There is no known cause for CRPS so to prove that a doctor caused it is extremely difficult. Even with that knowledge I decided to move forward.

Once the official paperwork was filed I was subpoenaed for an official deposition. I knew this would be part of the process, but I don't think anything can ever prepare you for it. First of all you are in the hot seat and you are made to feel like you are the one in the wrong. The questions are very intentional to break you down and try to find any flaw or any way to blunder your case. You do your best to stick to the, "yes" or "no" answers that your lawyer has asked you to give, but then they hit you with questions that require a detailed answer. There are no takebacks on a deposition and no do-overs.

I had an uphill battle from the beginning. Court filings, depositions, having the case postponed by the defendant's lawyers – over and over again. At one point my case was the longest standing malpractice case in Orange County. The judge was not too happy about that and neither was I.

During my journey with my doctors I was told many things and had many conversations. As a patient I assumed that people will be honest and truthful especially when under oath. I found out the hard way this is not always the case.

Since my lawyer had no way of knowing what was or was not said during previous doctor's appointments I was asked to sit in on all of the depositions regardless of whether we requested them or Dr. Hauser's lawyer's requested them. Sitting there I wasn't allowed to say a word while the deposition was going on, but I could send a note to my lawyer if something is out of context or wrong.

Reliving the doctor appointments, treatments, surgeries, pain and hell is not fun especially when you are still in the throes of it. Stress levels are extremely high and anxiety levels continue to increase every time you step into the room where a deposition is going to happen.

I remember feeling completely overwhelmed as I walked into the deposition that would involve Dr. Hauser. I wasn't sure I could sit through it as I was sure he would not tell the truth and there was nothing I could say. Tension was high that day on all sides. It was evident that he was not thrilled about being there and he certainly did not want to make eye contact with me. There were a lot of, "*I do not recall*" comments made and other answers that were skewed to fit his narrative. I was prepped ahead of time to expect this, but the emotions that come while sitting there and listening to someone so smugly answering questions is infuriating.

My lawyer knew it was a very emotional day for me. Instead of just leaving me on my own he opted for us to grab lunch to discuss the case, the deposition and to make sure I was ok. Every day he was learning more and more about CRPS and how it impacted my life.

The weeks turned into months and months turned into years as we slowly moved from deposition to deposition. Anyone that had ever treated me in the past was being subpoenaed and deposed. This was from Dr. Hauser's side not ours, but it could be utilized to our advantage if needed.

They were looking for a needle in a hay stack.

Anything that could possibly throw this case off track.

There are a couple of depositions that are seared into my memory. One is from the orthopedic foot and ankle surgeon that had to clean up after Dr. Hauser. He specifically told me, *"... it looked like a bomb went off in my foot, and told me the incision was made in the wrong place."* Yet when he was deposed there were a lot of, *"I don't recall"*, statements being made. On the way out of the room that day he walked by my side, looked around to make sure there was no one within ear shot and apologized. He said he just couldn't get involved and wished me the best.

I left there that day dumbfounded. I told my lawyer what happened and he said there was nothing that could be done. This is part of the problem with proving a malpractice case. You have to either have doctors that are willing to stand with you or you have to have some incredible experts.

We turned to the experts.

Listening to some experts is just not the best thing for a CRPS or chronic pain patient though. It can be very depressing to hear that the future is bleak and could be filled with unfathomable pain, suffering and possible loss of toes or limbs. I was in shock hearing this and I refused to believe what I was hearing. There was no way that I could allow my condition to progress to that point, to get anywhere near what was being described.

Each day dealing with my malpractice case brought more stress, anxiety and despair. Having to relive what I had already been through over and over again was not helping me to heal. It was actually making me worse.

The time had come to make a decision. Do I move forward with a jury trial and put my faith in the hands of people that knew nothing about CRPS or chronic pain. They will look at me and see someone walking into court with a cane but otherwise looking ok. They will look at a doctor and hear this skewed story. Who will they believe? If I lose I will have to pay all of Dr. Hauser's lawyer's fees, all of the deposition fees (there were tons) and the court costs. If I win the most I can get because of California state law for Medical Malpractice is $250,000 for pain and suffering. Even if the jury awards more the judge will change it to the maximum award of $250,000. This law has not changed since 1976.

There were many conversations and many sleepless nights about this. I finally decided that we would go ahead and move forward with mediation. I was not thrilled with not being able to get Dr. Hauser's medical license but I was to the point that I needed some closure with all of this. I was hopeful that I could say my peace to him face to face and walk away. Little did I know that he requested separate mediation rooms because he did not want to face me.

Preparations were made and the big day finally arrived. It was a very interesting process. Our mediator was a retired Judge and he knew all too well how hard it would have been to prove a case like this to a jury. The day drew on as he had to move between rooms to try to find a settlement and a happy medium. After 7 hours of tug-of-war an agreement was struck. I didn't get his license as I had hoped, but if another patient ever looked him up they would see the case and charges filed.

Prior to leaving the mediator came back in and asked permission to speak with me. He was very understanding of everything that I had been through and the road that I still had in front of me. He said in time as the laws change it will be easier to prove these type of cases in court, but right now it is still extremely difficult. He told me that he knew that there was still a lot of healing to do, but he hoped that I could move on and find solace in the future.

CHAPTER 13

Germany: Quest for Remission

Following the removal of my spinal cord stimulator there were many conversations with medical professionals, clinics, family members and friends. I was now on a quest to find a treatment that would allow me to dramatically decrease my pain, regain my life and preferably gain remission. I was a firm believer that where there was a will, there was a way.

I had a family member that had just returned from being treated at a private clinic in Germany, and while there she spoke to their Medical Director about my dilemma. She was surprised to hear that he was familiar with CRPS. In Germany it was referred to as Sudeck's Syndrome. He felt it was more of an autoimmune related condition and was confident he could help me.

Any glimmer of hope was worth a second look. I set up a time to Skype with their clinic to discuss my case, the treatments I had already gone through, and possible treatment options they could offer. The confidence exuded during my conversation put me at ease and it seemed that they had a game plan on how we could move forward. The biggest hurdle I had to get over was the extremely long flight from Los Angeles to Frankfurt, Germany. I knew that once I arrived I could adapt to just about anything.

A lot of thought and prayer was put into the decision to make the trip to Germany. I felt that this was the best option that I had in front of me at the time, so I started the preparation to move forward.

There was so much to do from plane tickets, medical records being sent to Germany, a quick follow up visit with Dr. Amir, and mentally preparing for what felt like potentially life changing trip.

The big day had arrived. I was excited and terrified at the same time. Several weeks post-op from having my spinal cord stimulator removed I was still healing. My CRPS was only being maintained with medication; which was taking the edge off the pain but that was about it.

My mother-in-law was going to fly back to Frankfurt with me as she had to redo a blood test that was only available there. It would be nice to have someone with me that was familiar with the lay of the land and to have emotional support.

We were flying out of Los Angeles International Airport (LAX) on a non-stop flight to Frankfurt. Arrangements had been made for wheelchair assistance through the airport both at LAX and in Frankfurt. Once we arrived they would have someone meet us at the airport to pick us up and take us to clinic and/or our flat (apartment). The wheels were in motion. Now all I had to do was endure the trip.

This was the first time I had flown since I had been diagnosed with my CRPS. I had never had wheelchair assistance before and I felt very awkward asking for it. On the other hand I knew that all the international flight were on the furthest side of the airport and with the long flight ahead I needed to take every precaution I could. There were a lot of jokes between my mother-in-law Dottie and myself to try to keep things light, but my mind continued to race as we got closer to boarding the flight.

The time had come to pre-board. I had never seen a plane this big in my life. It was enormous. We had a few extra minutes to find our seats and try to get situated prior to the flood of other passengers coming aboard. I had intentionally booked a window seat in hopes that I could somewhat protect my foot and ankle. This was a 12-hour flight. Having my foot down that length of time would definitely lead to additional swelling and pain.

Once we finally took off from Los Angeles the service on our flight was fantastic. I had all of my medications with me, headphones, books, magazines, etc. I didn't anticipate the entire flight being put to 'bed' heading over; so to say. About a third of the way into the flight everyone is instructed to lower their window shade, the lights are turned off and essentially the passengers on the plane are put to bed. It was the craziest thing I had seen, but then again this was the first transcontinental flight I had been on.

It was difficult to get comfortable especially with the areas in my back and hip that were still healing. Add in the spread of my CRPS from my left foot/ankle into those areas and I was dealing with a whole new cup of tea. Medication helped me to doze off and on, it was taking the edge off the pain, but I was anxious. I did the best I could to find some good movies to watch to try to take my mind off of my pain as the hours ticked away.

Finally, we arrived in Frankfurt. As everyone was hustling to collect their belonging to exit the plane we waited patiently. There were hundreds of passengers on board between the different levels of the plane, so it was like a city of ants all trying to move in one direction. Sometimes the best thing to do is to just sit back and wait for the commotion to stop so that you can proceed ahead safely.

I had an airport attendant waiting for me with a wheelchair to take us down to baggage claim. It wasn't quite that easy though since we were flying in from out of country. There were several stops that we had to make along the way. Yet having wheelchair assistance made each one of these stops much quicker and more efficient from everything I was told. Once our bags were finally obtained we went through customs and out to the unrestricted area of the airport to see a gentleman there holding a sign, "Traci Patterson".

Constantine would be my driver while I was there and a wealth of information. His wife, Angela, worked at the clinic as a Naturopathic doctor. What an amazing couple.

Dottie and I were delivered to the flat to start getting settled in. Our bags were brought up for us and we found a lovely basket of groceries there to greet us too. On the table was a local cell phone with the clinic number pre-programmed in. It wasn't more than an hour when the cell phone was ringing. It actually caught me off guard as I just wasn't expecting a call or to go anywhere that day. All I wanted to do was to elevate my foot and to rest, but they had other plans for me.

Two hours later we had a buzz at the door intercom. It was Constantine saying he was there to pick us up and take us to the clinic. On our way. Keep in mind it is January in Germany, yes this means winter time there and I cannot put a sock on my foot much less anything that is warm. Grabbing coats, scarves and out the door we go. The reality of the situation was starting to set in as we drove to the clinic. Here I was in a foreign country, a CRPS patient, I was hoping for a miracle, but the reality was I had no idea what I was getting into.

The staff greeted me as we arrived. Angela went back to finish up with another patient as I sat down to go over my case with the Medical Director. I filled out the necessary paperwork and we discussed where I was treatment wise and the removals of the stimulator. We started talking about some of the treatments that they wanted to do with me and how they would integrate more as we moved forward.

Part of their theory was CRPS tied into an auto-immune issue. Therefore, they wanted to work on 'modulating' my immune system. Detoxing to rid my body of excess toxins that had built up from years of medications and inflammation. Working on lymphatic drainage to help decrease swelling. I would use, Thymus Cell Therapy, to increase my own cell counts to do Stem Cell Therapy. This was autologous stem cell therapy utilizing my own blood, having my own stem cells harvested by a microbiologist and then grown in a lab. After a week I would have millions of my own stem cells. Ozone therapy, neural therapy, working with a personal trainer to increase muscle tone, etc.

I had no idea what to expect, but I knew I had to keep an open mind. I was there to do everything that I could to try to regain my life. This was a bit overwhelming. I was learning to go with the flow even when I just wanted to curl up in a ball in the corner.

We moved into a larger room for treatment to start. My heart was pounding even though this was probably the most laid back and comfortable setting I had ever been in for any type of treatment. I had a chaise instead of an uncomfortable exam table. This was a good start.

Then the dreaded reality hit. They needed to examine my foot and ankle to have an idea of where the CRPS started and ended. They were fascinated with the continually moving toe, but then again everyone had been. They also needed to examine my back and hip following the stimulator surgeries and progression of the CRPS. Knowing how painful it was, they were as gentle as possible. I kept telling myself this was all necessary to make progress.

Next came something I had not expected, Neural Therapy. *Neural therapy is a method of diagnosing and treating illness and pain caused by disturbances of the body's electrophysiology. These electrical disturbances, called "interference fields," are manifestations of cell membrane instability and typically trigger abnormal autonomic nervous system responses. Interference fields may be found in scars, autonomic ganglia, teeth, internal organs or other locations where local tissue irritation exists. [http://www.neuraltherapybook.com/NTdefined.php]*

It was explained to me that they would inject Procaine into the scars on my ankle and foot where they did the surgeries and then follow these injections with Ozone. The purpose is to break any 'interference fields' and to stabilize the autonomic nervous system (ANS). Well, in theory this made sense and it is a treatment protocol that is used quite a bit in Germany. One big concern I had prior to starting was that I could barely touch my foot; much less my scars from my surgery; so how did they plan on injecting these areas? I was told it was a very fine needle – as they prepped to start.

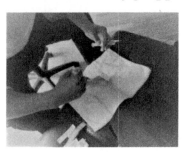

The room was absolutely silent when we started. I swear you could have heard a pin drop. I was afraid to breath. I had so many memories of painful injections free flowing through my head. It was one awful thought after another and we had not even started yet. I knew I had to do whatever it took to stop and concentrate on a good outcome. It was time to start with the upper medial scar and then move through the other three scars that were on my ankle and foot. He let me know he was ready to start and I watched the first injection puncture the skin, the very corner of the scar and it was the most horrific pain that I had experienced in my life. The worst part was it was only the first injection! I yelped in pain as I just could not hold it in as tears were rolling down my face. Each injection of Procaine only added to the immense pain that I was already feeling. It was an accumulative affect at this point. I was wondering how much I could really take at one time. Finally we finished the Procaine injections. Sigh, breath... But, now we had to do the Ozone injections in the exact area that he just did injected with Procaine. Holly crap! There was no way that I could do this.

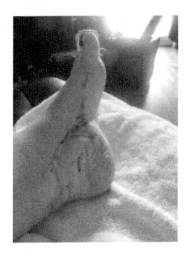

Everyone sat there telling me it would be ok and to just hang in there as I was yelping like a dog that had just been hit by a car. My heart was racing, my face and chest were red and blotchy, and I thought I was going to pass out because the pain was so bad. When we finally finished with Neural Therapy they left me alone for a few minutes to try to recover.

The Medical Director came back in to do some Ozone Therapy. This consisted of additional Ozone Therapy externally with my left foot/ankle and blood Ozone Therapy. I have to say that I got a kick out of the blood Ozone Therapy as it is like a reverse IV. You have an IV started, the tourniquet is left on and a glass IV bottle is utilized. This glass bottle is slowly filled with your blood and then they add ozone to it. Once it is the correct mixture then the tunicate is removed and the blood-ozone mixture is returned to the body. Fascinating.

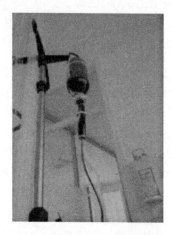

We wrapped up with an IV and then an injection with Thymus Cell Therapy. I was exhausted, overwhelmed and in pain. I had come this far so I had to trust the process, but at this point I just wanted to get back to the flat.

We headed out and there was another patient there being treated for breast cancer. She needed to be dropped off at her flat too. Then it dawned on me that she had the pleasure of hearing me while I was doing the Neural Therapy. I was so embarrassed. I tried to make a joke out of it and told her that if she heard all the commotion I was sorry. She was great and let me know that she completely understood and there was no reason to apologize for anything. It was never brought up again.

Constantine dropped us at the flat and made sure we knew when he would be by to pick us up in the morning. Apparently parking was awful and it was better to wait for him curbside if possible.

I was thankful to have my mother-in-law there. She fixed dinner that evening and made sure that things were taken care of. I was so spent from the flight over, little sleep, stress, anxiety and the treatments that day that I just wanted to collapse. I was able to get in a quick nap before dinner. Then we made our Skype calls home to discuss the events of the day, and finally off to bed.

The next morning seemed to come quickly. I was dealing with jet lag, my pain levels were still high, and I was stressed out and anxious about what was to come. On top of that we had two females trying to get ready in a rather small bathroom at the same time. We managed to get through the morning routine and even get a quick Skype call home prior to leaving to meet Constantine.

We were met with a lot of traffic heading in and had to stop to pick up the patient we met yesterday. I was so used to having to be punctual for all of my appointments, but this was a bit different since it was their driver and we were now on their schedule. Allowing myself to let go of controlling the situation was a bit of a hurdle. I did the best I could to just take in the Main River, the skyline of Frankfurt and the awe of actually being in Germany.

Finally we arrived at the clinic and made our way in. We were all greeted and offered some fresh green juice, water and/or coffee. They wanted to know how the night went and then it was a matter of jumping into the planned treatments. We talked about continuing with the Neural Therapy and adding in my back and hip incisions/scars from the stimulators. Ozone Therapy, IV's, and Thymus Cell Therapy would all be a consistent regimen. In the next day or so we would add in some type of PT or training to try to get my body moving again. Then introduce lymphatic massage to help decrease inflammation. I would have an appointment the following week to have my blood drawn for my Stem Cell Therapy, but we would talk more about that later.

With the pleasantries over it was time to get down to business. Neural Therapy was first on the to-do-list. I really wanted to just throw in the towel when I realized that this would be done every single day. Yesterday has horrific and that is an understatement. Yet, here I am in Germany seeking treatment, a way to get better, so I just felt like I was backed into a corner and had to do whatever it took to move forward. Even neural therapy.

I started out on a padded treatment table closer to the windows. We would start with the scars on my ankle/foot and then move to the scars on my back and hip. Let the fun begin.

My mother-in-law came over to stand by my side in case I needed her as we started. I watched as the first syringe filled with Procaine was prepped and the first injection was made. As soon as the needle touched my foot and punctured the skin a sharp, intense electrical pain radiated through my body. Just as the day before a yelp instantly came out and tears were rolling down my face. Dottie grabbed my hand to try to comfort me but when the second and subsequent injections were done I squeezed so hard that I just about broke the hand that was trying to support me. She was cringing in pain from her hand and I was writhing in pain with every injection. Finally we finished with my ankle/foot. They were getting ready to start on my back as I was trying to talk them into skipping my back until the following day. They weren't buying into what I had to say and kept telling me it was necessary to help me. We did the same procedure of Procaine and Ozone into the scars from the stimulator surgeries. The whole clinic seem so quiet except for my squeals, yelps and sobs as I dug into the pillow on my lap. Yes, I switched out a hand for a pillow. By the time we finally finished I was shaking, felt flush and was completely overwhelmed. They gave me a blanket and asked me to lie down for a bit. All I could think was, "*Is this going to get any easier?*"

After I finally stopped shaking, I felt like I was gaining some composure. If this is what torture felt like then I completely understood why it was so horrific and people died from it. I had millions of thoughts running through my head about whether I had made the right decision to come here, but I knew I had to try to focus on the outcome that I wanted.

We were about to resume treatment so I moved over to the chaise and we picked up with the Ozone Therapy. I was just fascinated with how blood ozone therapy worked. It was a good way to distract me from my pain. This was followed with a couple of IVs. While one of the IV's was running I met with Angela to do a lymphatic massage. I had so much swelling throughout my body that we needed to do something to try to try to reset my body. This was followed up with the Thymus Cell Therapy to increase my cell counts and then we were done for the day.

We were driven back to our flat and I was more than ready to rest. We quickly realized that we needed some groceries though. I was in no condition physically or emotionally to walk down to the store after the day that I just had, so Dottie grabbed a couple of bags and headed out. We just needed the fixings for dinner and breakfast. Then we would have them drive us to a grocery store the following day.

While Dottie was gone I tried to get as comfortable as possible and grabbed a quick nap.

That night was filled with anxiety on my part, interesting conversations, Skype video chats home and trying to pass time with finding channels on German television we could understand or that were in English. I turned in early as Dottie worked on the computer.

I was up early the next morning. I took advantage of the bank of windows overlooking the street below. It was nice to people watch, take in a different culture and try to distract my mind. Across the street was a little store that reminded me of a little corner store that you would find in the US that carried a little bit of everything. They had a small sidewalk café, newspapers, nickknacks, and necessities. Perhaps we could drop in there later in the day if I felt up to it.

Dottie and I were getting settled into a routine. We knew what time we would be picked up and where to meet. From there we would pick up the other patient on our way in to the clinic and jump into the treatment protocols.

Today they had a bit of a surprise for me at the

clinic. Jorg came in to meet me. He was a personal trainer. He worked with a company that had a very unique approach to training that involved a vest with electrodes and other straps that went around the biceps, quads and glutes. As they were trying to explain this to me I was a bit hesitant, but it had to be better than Neural Therapy.

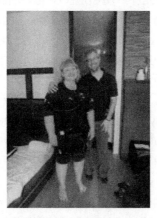

Once suited up we started out the session out lying on the matt/bed area. Jorg was learning English and I did not know German/Deutsch so we utilized his i-Pad to learn common words. Jorg would turn on a specific region then increase the intensity until I told him it was enough. The electrodes in the vest or on the other areas mentioned would cause the muscle(s) to contract based upon the signal sent. While this was happening he would give me a specific exercise or movement to do. The two things combined were amazing.

By the end of our session I had learned a few key

words in Deutsch and Jorg was learning more English. I was the first chronic pain or CRPS patient that he had ever worked with here. Things went well and I was looking forward to my next session with him.

Now it was time to change back into my clothes and get mentally prepared for Neural Therapy. Today was no different than the previous days except I knew what to expect. The injections were just as painful and I did everything I could to try to breathe through the pain. Today I even brought my i-pod and tried listening to a relaxation mp3 file to take my mind off what was happening. Unfortunately, the intense pain associated with needles stabbing into scars that were in the middle of my CRPS over road anything that I tried to accomplish with keeping my composure. Two injections in and I had tears streaming down my face. By the third injection all bets were off and I had yelps and squeals coming out with each and every injection. Just as with the previous day by the time we finished my ankle, foot, back and hip I was shaking like a leaf, felt cold and clammy, and I honestly felt like my body was going into shock.

After I had the opportunity to recuperate a bit from the Neural Therapy then we pick up with the Ozone Therapy, IV's and Thymus Cell Therapy. During the remaining treatments I kept telling myself that this would get better, I would survive and I would get better. I knew inside that ultimately the pieces would come together.

Today we were going shopping following my treatments. We needed to get groceries for the flat and it was easier to accomplish that if they took us. I was slowly learning key words that were important for groceries, shopping, and some areas of the body.

We got help bringing up our groceries. Once everything was put away I wanted to go over to the little store across the street. I thought I saw something in their front window and I wanted to check it out in person. Dottie and I donned our jackets and headed out. We were checking things out for little souvenirs to take back home but I did indeed see a stuffed hippopotamus in the front window. Dottie looked at me funny but at this point she played along. We got the hippo and a couple of other little items. If nothing else the hippo put a smile on my face, and it would give me something to squish while they were doing the Neural Therapy.

I was tired as it had been a long day.

The rest of the week was much of the same routine: Neural Therapy, Ozone Therapy, IV's, lymphatic massage and Thymus Cell Therapy. They got a laugh out of my hippo but fully understood that it was better to have something to squeeze than to break someone's hand. As a matter of fact they named the hippo Hanne.

As the week progressed I started to get out of the flat a bit more. On Saturday we all met - the staff and patients - to go to the Konstablerwache farmers market. All of the local farmers and merchants bring in their vegetables, fruits, flowers, cheese, brats, beer and more. It was wonderful. The sights and smells. I was trying to enjoy it as much as possible as I carefully worked my way through the crowds with my cane. We sat to enjoy a lunch of German brats and refreshments in the middle of the hustle and bustle. It was quite the place.

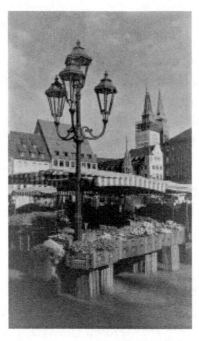

Everyone wanted to go shopping after lunch. This was the most I had done in years and I was just not up to it. My CRPS was letting me know that I was pushing the envelope and I was afraid to undo any potential progress that I was starting to make. Instead of everyone ending their day early to drive me back to the flat I said it would be just as easy to grab a taxi. My mother-in-law, Dottie, opted to go back with me. Prior to leaving we were reminded that everything would be closed on Sunday. So, if there was anything else that we needed this would be the time to get it.

Coming from the US where we are used to having access to everything 24/7 this was indeed a change. In Germany they take Sunday as a day off. The grocery stores are closed, department stores, gas stations, malls, etc. they are all closed. The only things that are open will be a handful of restaurants and the tourist areas. This is why we were reminded to make sure that we had what we needed for Sunday.

Our day of rest, Sunday, was uneventful. We decided to take a small walk that morning to get out and grab some fresh air. A few blocks down the street we found a small bakery that happened to be open to our surprise. It was a popular place. The aroma wafting out the door just lured you in. We did our best to communicate with pointing then asking if they spoke English as we grabbed a couple of croissants and goodies for later. Our return trek to the flat was a bit slower but I was impressed with myself that I managed to do it. This was saying something.

Ah, it was Monday. It had come so quickly. It was time for my treatments to begin again and to see what would happen next. For the most part every day had a routine by now. I guess you could say that we were getting into a groove. As for myself there was a lot packed in - treatment wise - in a 4 hour period, but other than the Neural Therapy it was all pretty relaxed.

Constantine picked us up to make our drive in to the clinic. Traffic was unusually congested today because there was a partial transit strike over wages. Therefore, there were more people driving and on bikes than they were used to. A large majority of people use mass transit in Germany. It is easy and is cost effective. So, when there is a strike or partial strike it dramatically effects your ability to get from point A to point B.

Our detours and side streets allowed me to see areas of Frankfurt that I may not have been able to have seen otherwise. We kept Constantine busy with questions and pulling information about points of interest during our commute. It was quite informative and interesting.

When we finally arrived at the clinic I was debriefed about the weekend, how did I feel, were there any changes, etc. I think we were all pleasantly happy about our outing on Saturday and Sunday, and the fact that there was not a huge flare following either day. We all agreed that was progress. This week would pretty much follow the same routine except for one day that would be set aside to drive up to see Dr. Pesic to draw my blood for the stem cells to be harvested, grown and then in a week I would have millions of my own stem cells.

Neural Therapy never got any easier. There were some days that it was decided that we would split up treating my ankle/foot and back/hip. Combined it was overload on my system and every time I had the exact same reaction of feeling like my body was going into shock.

Jorg came back for another session with the 'electric vest'. This was something that I actually looked forward to. It gave me some ability to feel like I had control over what I was doing. Plus, I felt like I was getting a little stronger with each session I did with Jorg.

Midway through the week we - the Medical Director, the CEO, Dottie and I - took an hour plus drive to Dr. Pesic's office in Bad Harzburg. It was an honor meeting him as he actually did the stem cells for President Ronald Regan. Today they just needed to draw 25+ vials of blood so that my stem cells could be harvested and then grown by their microbiologist. This was easier said than done. Did I ever mention that I have awful veins? Dr. Pesic started with trying to do a blood draw from my left arm and that didn't work. Then he moved to another vein and that didn't work. Next was my hand and that didn't work. I felt like a human pin cushion. Hot compresses, hot packs, every trick was pulled out of the hat to make this work. Finally the Medical Director came in to try to make a go of it. He had been doing IVs on me since I arrived so I was confident that he would have better luck.

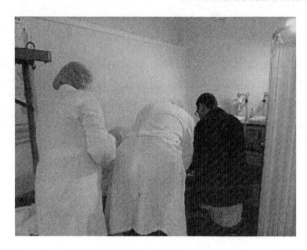

Thankfully, he did have better luck and they were able to start accumulating the blood necessary to move forward with the stem cell process. In total they drew approximately 30 vials of blood that day. I was left with many bruises and blown veins, but if the outcome was anything like what we discussed it would be worth it.

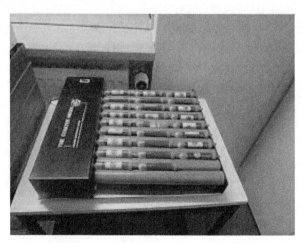

Following all the poking, prodding and praying I was left under a warm blanket to recover while, "Das Original" band-aides were put all over me. I was sure that they would run out of band-aides prior to finishing.

Rather than heading straight back they decided to take us on a small sightseeing detour. This was a nice break.

We stopped at Eckertal. This is a hamlet on the eastern rim of Bad Harzburg. Eckertal was an area during the post-war division of Germany where there was an inner Germany border. On November 11, 1989 around 4:30pm the highway was re-opened between Eckertal and Stapelburg. From a historic point of view this was the first border crossing between the East and West Germany in the process of reunification. We were able to see the monument that had been erected at the site.

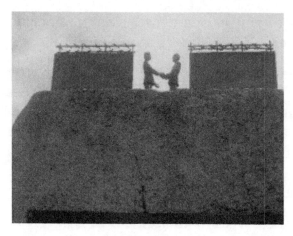

From there we drove over to a nearby village that was just amazing. It reminded you of something out of a fairytale or movie. The large towers and turrets, old mid-century churches, and cobblestone streets. It was difficult to take it all in. It was cold, there were a few snowflakes beginning to fall and I had no socks on, only Crocs, and didn't even have a coat on. I didn't expect to go on an outing so I was not prepared.

We did some window shopping, took in the sights and had some laughs prior to heading back. Everyone else could have spent several more hours there but I was worn out. It had been a long day for me.

The following week came quick enough. Every day seemed to be flying by. I was seeing a slight decrease in my pain and I was able to walk a bit further each day. This was good news.

It didn't matter what I did or how I tried to prepare myself, Neural Therapy never got any easier. Breathing, music, distractions, yelling, squealing... nothing seemed to make that portion of my treatment plan any easier. Bottom line was if it could help me get better then I was willing to do whatever it took.

I looked forward to Jorg coming in. This was something different that I could tell was helping me get stronger. The time with Jorg and working with the 'electric suit' was a good distraction. Not only was it a time of learning, it was a time of encouragement, and seeing that I could get stronger. All in all this played a huge part in my physical and emotional wellbeing.

Midweek we would drive back up to Dr. Pesic's office to have my stem cells injected back into me. This was exciting. I knew there was no magic wand that could undo everything, but the stem cells made sense and seemed like a very plausible solution. Everyone kept impressing on me that to see the full effects of the stem cells it could take up to 6 months. It would not be an overnight solution.

We had a good drive up to Dr. Pesic and the injection of my stem cells was so much easier than the numerous needle sticks and drawing all the vials of blood. Following the injection (over a million of my own stem cells) I was asked to rest for a bit. I didn't see or feel any different following the injection. I was just hoping and praying for a good outcome. With hugs all around we left to head back to Frankfurt.

As the week progressed I was more optimistic about having a positive outcome. For the first time in years I actually fell asleep with my feet touching. Now this may not sound like a big deal to others, but when you have been dealing with so much pain that anything that touches your foot sends you into a tail spin it is huge. It got me thinking that I had 1 week left here. I was questioning if I needed to stay longer and if it would even be possible. At this point I could do an extra week by myself.

I brought up this up with the Medical Director. I wanted to know in his opinion if I were to stay an extra week or two did he think I would gain anything from it. As expected the answer was, yes, they felt that by staying an additional week or two that I would only continue to decrease my pain levels. With this news I had a big decision to make. I needed to speak with my family, check on extending, and really think and pray about this decision.

My mother-in-law, Dottie, had committed to coming with me for the three week stent. I didn't expect her to stay longer if I decided to extend my stay. Knowing this could potentially be a burden on her, the last thing that I wanted was to impose. This was about healing and finding a way forward.

That evening I called a friend and confidant back in the US. I was in a quandary. My gut was telling me I needed to stay for an extra week to see how much relief I could get, but I was feeling pressure to go home. I didn't want to cross lines with anyone, but this trip had to be about me and not anyone else at this point. I felt like my life was hanging by a thread and this decision could ultimately dictate my future. We had a good conversation and it was reiterated to me that I needed to listen to my gut instinct. It was nice to have outside support even if we were across the globe from each other.

The next day I spoke with staff at the clinic to find out what I would need to do to extend my stay. As it turned out it would be easier than expected. They would contact the airline on my behalf and let them know due to a medical necessity I needed to extend my ticket and they would extend my housing. In the long run Dottie decided to stay the extra time with me. So, things were moving forward, plans were in place, and now all I had to do was endure my remaining time and focus on healing.

The remaining weeks went by quickly. My days started get into a set routine of breakfast, morning pick up, casual drive to clinic, 3-4 hours of treatments, back to the flat, lunch, nap, walk, Skype, etc. A routine was just fine. I knew what to expect and I could tell that my stress levels had dropped while I was here.

As the time progressed I could feel my pain levels dropping. This was huge and a big lift for me. Especially when I allowed myself to think about what I was told following the removal of my spinal cord stimulator. I felt like there was no hope (at least for a few days) and my doctors had nothing more to offer. Now look at me. I actually have a smile on my face and my pain levels are going down.

I was anxious and excited to get back home. I was missing my family, but I was very anxious about what the future would hold. I was told the stem cells would continue to help regenerate my nerves in the coming months yet there was still a huge question on how to move forward especially since I was not completely pain free. Yes, my pain levels had dropped by several points and I was functioning. This didn't stop the questions and 'what if' in my mind.

My four weeks in Frankfurt were coming to an end. Today was my last day of treatment in the morning and then later in the afternoon we would catch our flight back to California. My pain levels were hovering around a 5/10 which was fantastic compared to when I arrived. The theory was that my pain levels should continue to diminish as the stem cells continue to work over the next 6 months. We also discussed utilizing supplements (Alpha Lipoic Acid, Turmeric, Magnesium, Vitamin C, etc.) to help.

Everything was packed up the night prior so there wouldn't be a huge rush that day. We were taken to the Frankfurt airport and got checked into our Lufthansa flight. Now the fun would begin was we headed off for another 12+ hour flight. I felt better about the flight going home then I did the flight heading over, but I was still a little anxious. I was worried about possible swelling in my ankle/foot with this long of a flight. I was concerned that someone may accidently step on my foot and undo any progress that I had made. There were many thoughts going through my mind, but I knew that I needed to stay as positive as possible.

Relieved and exhausted when we finally landed. I was ready to get home.

CHAPTER 14

Transcontinental Search for Answers

I was home for a couple months with my pain levels holding around 4-5/10. I was feeling pretty good about things until out of the blue I started to have coloration changes again and my pain levels started to slowly increase. Nothing had changed since I got home. I was following up with my pain management doctor, taking my meds as prescribed, taking the additional supplements and just trying to move forward. At first I thought it was a fluke, but as days turned into weeks and weeks turned into months I realized I had a problem.

Emails followed by Skype calls were made to Germany. What was I supposed to do at this point? All I knew was that I could not live my life in constant 24/7 pain that was off the charts. It was overwhelming and a huge setback. It was decided that I would return to Germany in June. On one hand this gave me a little comfort knowing I had an option but on the other hand I remembered how painful Neural Therapy had been and that was scary.

Soon enough the time came and I was on my way to Frankfurt again. This time I would make the trip on my own. I knew everyone at the clinic, I had my laptop to Skype home and I knew I could do it.

One big thing we were looking at this time was the incision/scar where my spinal cord stimulator was removed. It seemed to be getting more and more painful and there was a concern about the possibility of something besides CRPS causing this. I had an ultrasound done to the area where my stimulator was removed and sure enough they saw something was inside my back. With further discussions I gave permission to do a minor surgical procedure to open up the incision. None of us had any idea what we may find, but there was a lot of curiosity.

Yes, I was curious as to what was in my back but I also remembered that many medication were no longer working on me. Marcaine and lidocaine really didn't do a lot to numb or block areas. This scared me. How were they going to re-open the incision on my back? Here we go again. My head was filled with thousands of thoughts – most were not positive.

They tried to make it as easy as possible. Numbing the areas with a local anesthetic (procaine) and then utilizing a scalpel to dissect back each layer of the fascia. I tried to lay as still as possible while all of this was going on. Honestly, I was afraid to move.

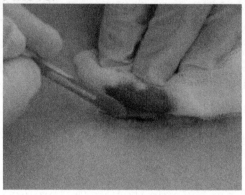

The Medical Director was explaining what was happening as he proceeded which was helpful. Each step of the way asking how I was doing. It wasn't too long before I was hearing that he found what looked like a piece of gauze that was left in the area. I was close to six months post op, so what was coming out was somewhat broken down. It was decided to leave the area open to heal on its own. They would check it daily and make sure it was healing properly.

Sigh...

I was really praying that this was the cause of the pain in and around the incision. I wanted that to be the solution and for this not to be CRPS. Unfortunately, that was not the case. CRPS had already crept into my back and taking out the gauze didn't change that. In fact I was dealing with it from my waist to my shoulders.

I would continue with much the same treatment plan as my previous trip minus Stem Cell Therapy. They did add in a couple of other items including ionization and procaine IVs in hopes that it would help calm down the nerves.

Neural therapy was a daily treatment and just as last time there was no getting used to it. No matter how prepared I thought I was going into it I was unprepared for the sheer pain it caused. I brought back Hanne the hippo to help me through this particular treatment. If nothing else she was something to squeeze to the point of no return. Every single day that I had to go through this I wondered if it was really worth it. I questioned my own sanity and what I was doing.

This was a short trip this time. I had set up three weeks to see what we could do. I was hopeful with some booster treatments that we could not only get my pain levels back to a 4-5/10 but maybe lower.

During this trip I so wanted to be independent. I wanted to be normal again, but when I pushed too hard my CRPS pushed back. I did take a day trip on the Main River which was a nice change of pace one weekend. While grabbing a taxi and heading to downtown on other days that I had time. I was slowly figuring out how to pace myself and I knew that it was easy to grab a taxi back to my flat if needed.

After the 3 weeks we wrapped up my treatment in Frankfurt. This trip had a completely different feel to it as there was more hustle and bustle at the clinic, more patients and they were in a new location. My pain levels did decrease down to a 4/10 and the incision on my back was closed. It was time to head home again.

As I packed I noticed that I was anxious and started to stress out. I hoped and prayed for the best outcome possible and wanted my pain levels to hold or continue to diminish. Yet at the same time my mind kept going back to all the times where things went wrong, to my last trip where my pain levels increased and it scared the crap out of me. What if this happened again? I tried to shake off the thoughts as I double checked to make sure that everything was packed but it was difficult.

Next stop, California.

The following week I had a follow-up appointment with my pain management doctor. I was excited to share that my pain levels were down again.

Dr. Amir walked into the room with his normal smile and greeting. He wanted to know what had been happening and how I was doing. I had mentioned that I just arrived back from Germany again, so he wanted to know what we did. As I filled him in on the treatments, different protocols, etc. Dr. Amir was busy Googling many of the things to try to see what exactly I did. It was a cat and mouse conversation of who could keep up with who as he was putting notes into the computer. He was happy that I was doing better, but I could tell that he was skeptical too.

Then I got to the part about the ultrasound and the area where my spinal cord stimulator was removed. He was in disbelief that it was even possible. As a matter of fact everything came to a complete halt in the exam room for a couple minutes that seemed like an eternity. I finally asked why I would make up something like that and he responded by telling me there was no reason I would. I disclosed that I knew this type of conversation would happen and that is exactly why they actually took picture during the procedure. That included taking out the gauze. I reiterated that I wasn't looking to place blame but I thought he should know why that particular incision/scar had continued to bother me. It didn't change the fact that I still had CRPS in my back, but it did diminish the additional pain I was dealing with in that specific incision.

Dr. Amir was intrigued by the treatment that I did in Germany and how they decreased my pain levels. I asked about trying to do some of them here, but they were not FDA approved treatments so that was impossible.

Over the next couple of months my pain levels again started to increase. It didn't seem to matter what I did or what supplements I took it was just happening. The anguish and frustration that came with this was just indescribable. I felt like my life was unraveling before my very eyes.

I had been in touch with the Medical Director from Germany to see if there was anything that I could possibly do here in California. I wanted to see what my options were. It may be possible to do some Procaine IVs here at an Integrative Medicine facility that I had been to a few times. He had done some consulting with this clinic and could give them the proper ratios if they were willing to do the IVs. Perhaps that could help. Something had to give me some relief.

The information was relayed to the Integrative Medicine facility here - proper ratios, how fast the IV should run, etc. Then I set up a schedule to start the Procaine IV regimen to see if it would help. While at their facility I also met with a clinician that worked with essential oils. She was able to do a custom blend of essential oils that she felt would help with my pain.

Over the next month my focus was on doing everything I could to control and drop my pain levels. This included physical therapy, essential oils, IVs, prescription medications, and supplements.

The other options would be to try to coordinate a trip down to Mexico. He was helping to oversee protocols being put into place at a clinic in Mexico and could coordinate treatments for me there if that would help.

There was a lot to process and a lot of decisions to make. I kept wondering why I couldn't find something here in the US that would help but I was just bumping up against so many walls, but I wasn't willing to give up.

I thought about my options, spoke with my family and did a lot of praying. At the time the most reasonable options seemed to be going down to Mexico. It was just a couple hour drive to the border, and I was told they could have a driver pick me up and take me down to the facility from there.

Once again I felt like my back was against a wall. I needed something to drop my pain levels and hopefully get me closer to regaining my life. I was bumping into walls with my research here in the US, so if there was even a glimmer of home by going to Mexico I was going to do it. We coordinated a time for me to head down there for a week to start.

I had a driver from the facility in Mexico meet me in San Diego. From there we drove back across the border. It was an easy drive and my driver made sure that my needs were met during our trek. When we arrived at the facility it was set up as a compound. It had security and was surrounded by a privacy fence. Once inside it was beautiful and immaculate. I wasn't sure what to expect, but this exceeded my expectations, at least on the surface.

I was greeted by their staff and checked in. Typically their patients stay on site and everything is provided for them. Once checked in I was met by their Administrator, nutritionist and a doctor for an evaluation of my case.

My initial conversation with the doctor and staff gave me the impression that I was the first CRPS patient that they had dealt with. I knew that they were receiving a treatment plan based upon my previous treatment in Germany so I felt a bit better. On the flip side I felt like a fish out of water because I was not on their normal itinerary which interrupted the flow both for them and for me.

On the positive side this was a medical compound that was overlooking the ocean with the most amazing views. It was meant as a place to rest, de-stress and allow your health needs to be taken care of.

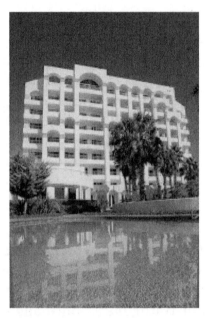

This week was full of a diverse set of treatments that were both familiar and new. They had the same regional hyperthermia machine that was in Germany, so I would do continual treatments of regional hyperthermia the entire week. They also wanted to add in HBOT, IPT (Insulin Potenti-ated Therapy), PK Protocol, Rife, Acuscope, Alpha

Lipoic and Myer Cocktail IVs, Chiropractic and nutrition. It was a very full week of treatments.

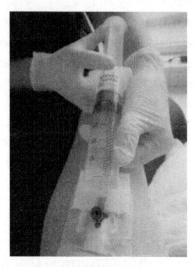

IPT was not what I had expected. This is a treatment that is typically used with cancer patients to allow for a very small dose of chemotherapy to be given, but in my case they used it with pain medication. When it was initially explained I had a lot of trepidation about it.

IPT uses insulin to increase the permeability of cell membranes in cells in order to increase the absorbance of therapeutic agents. When used to treat pain in conjunction with pain medication in IPT treatments, a dose of insulin is injected into a vein followed by a low dose of pain medication when the insulin has been absorbed. The pain medication dose is usually 10% to 25% of the traditionally prescribed dose. Then sugar water is injected to stop the hypoglycemia (low blood sugar) caused by the insulin injection.

My trepidation was something that was warranted. The first day of my IPT was not pleasant. I will be the first to admit that I have awful veins, and it is necessary to have an IV running during this process. It took many tries to even get an IV started. Then during the treatment they are administering insulin to decrease your glucose level to the point that you are hypoglycemic. There is a very small window in which the medication needs to be administered and then your blood sugar needs to be increased again. In my first go at this there was a miscommunication and a delay in pushing the pain medication and that resulted in a further delay in increasing my blood sugar levels. This delay left me at a very critical level and it took several hours to stabilize me following this procedure. Physically and mentally I felt awful.

My week continued with the coordination of treatments and the staffing doing their best to help in whatever way they could.

Another day of IPT was coming up and I could just feel my blood pressure rising. After my first experience with it I was extremely leery of doing it again. I was assured it would be ok and this could be a good way of controlling my pain.

Feeling like my back was against a wall, again we moved forward with the IPT. Monitors were started, after several attempts an IV was placed and the process began. The lower your glucose goes the worse you feel and the more out of it you become. Then as luck would have it my IV blew. It was a mad rush to start another IV as my glucose levels continued to drop. I just remember the doctors and nurses yelling in Spanish rather than English as things got tense. Finally after several unsuccessful tries an IV was placed, the pain medication was pushed and glucose followed. The blown IV caused my glucose levels to drop lower than they should have gone and this resulted in a long stay in recovery while they stabilized me.

Any other treatments planned for that day had just been thrown out the window. But, I learned a long time ago that you have to go with the flow. Take the good with the bad and learn to bounce back.

The week was filled with ups and downs - smiles and tears - and the hope that one of the many treatments would trigger something in my body to get me pain free. Getting pain free didn't happen but lowering my pain level did.

Back home once again I continued with my routine. Following up with my Pain Management doctor, taking pain medications, supplements, utilizing essential oils and anything else that I could think of. Yet like clockwork my pain levels started to increase again within a very short period of time.

This setback was more than a disappointment. How many times could a person have to go through the highs and lows? How much could I actually go through? This threw me into an emotional downward spiral.

I wasn't able to be there for my family or son the way I wanted to be. I felt like the biggest loser on earth. How was I supposed to move forward if I didn't feel like I had a life worth living? Would it be easier on everyone if I wasn't a burden anymore? It would be easy enough with all of the medications I had access to, but what would happen to my family? What example would I be setting for my son if I just threw in the towel? Millions of horrific thoughts were twirling in my head, but common sense won out. I always told everyone else, "*Where there is a will, there is a way.*" So, it was time to practice what I had been preaching.

Once again calls were made, emails were sent and I had to decide what to do. Over the next six months to a year I continued treatment out of country. I made two more trips to Germany and two more trips to Mexico all in hopes of regaining my life.

These trips were filled with much of the same treatments that I had done previously and we added in some new twists to try to shake things up a bit. It didn't seem to matter what we did as nothing was holding long-term. It was a vicious cycle that was physically, emotionally and spiritually draining.

CHAPTER 15

Mind Body Medicine for Healing

Prior to my last trip to German I had been referred to a Master Hypnotist that specialized in pain management. He was highly regarded for his background in working with pain patients. I didn't jump at the opportunity because I had been seen by someone locally doing hypnosis early on and it didn't work. Therefore, why would this be any different?

I spoke with Ron on the phone and sent several emails back and forth prior to deciding to see him. While emails were flowing, and discussions were happening I was finishing up my last trip to Germany. The treatments, specifically Neural Therapy, were overwhelming and I just wasn't sure how much more I could actually take.

During that trip I sent an urgent email asking for help. Hoping Ron could refer me to someone in Germany or do a telehealth session with me to help. Unfortunately, I had no luck on either side. Neural therapy left me a bit traumatized and the long-term outcomes just weren't there from either Germany or Mexico. It was time to seriously look at another option.

I was intrigued and skeptical at the same time about using hypnosis. How was this going to work when I had tried everything else? Yet, in my heart I knew that I could not leave one stone unturned. I had to give it a go.

I contacted Ron once again for possible treatment. After speaking we set up a time to be seen mid-November, 2013. I was told that it would be a week-long intensive that would include our time together and homework each evening (i.e. reading, listening to CD's, etc.). Compared to everything I had been through this was exciting and I was dedicated to get the most out of everything.

The trip to his office was well planned but still wore on me. It took two flights and a 45-minute drive to get to my final destination. My travel day only increased my stress and pain, but I knew I had to have an open mind.

Morning came early as there was a three hour time difference. I had no idea what to expect or what would happen later that day. I just knew that I needed to be as positive as possible and try to get as much out of this as I could. Downstairs they provided breakfast at the hotel, so I made a stop there prior to heading over to the office.

Arriving in the parking lot that was across from their building I just sat in my car for what seemed like an eternity. My mind was flipping through all of the treatments, the procedures, surgeries, and not so good outcomes that led me to this point. Finally, I realized that I just needed to set my thoughts aside for the time being and trust.

The first day was an eye opener. Learning more about the neuro-net of the brain, the limbic system, and how these played a large role in the chronic pain loop. This actually made sense, and made more sense than many of the treatments that I had gone through up to this point. We discussed changing 'pain levels' to 'comfort levels', so the brain focuses on it differently.

While working together the first day, it was discovered that I was also dealing with a case of PTSD due to everything that I had dealt with over the years. The treatments, being given medications for anesthesia and not having them work – then being able to feel everything during procedures, being told over and over there was nothing more that could be done, going through some treatments that were extremely uncomfortable, and negative comments from physicians about the possible outcome of my situation. This did not surprise me to say the least.

Over the week we used a combination of:

Clinical Hypnosis
Imagery and Visualizations
Neuroplasticity Training
Biofeedback
Light/Sound Therapy
"Issue Solution Training"
Learning Self-Hypnosis and more.

Throughout the week I saw progress. Some days it seemed like baby steps, but I was determined that this had to work.

The other huge thing that Ron was able to assist me with was a continual spasm or uncontrollable motor deficiency in the little toe on my left foot. This was in addition to my CRPS, and it was due to a nicked Lateral Plantar Nerve. I had many doctors consult with me regarding this, and I was always told that they had never seen anything like it. They had no idea what to do. Thus, I had been living with my little toe being in continual spams since 2006, and in 3 days, we were able to get my little toe to stop moving. Wow, this was a mechanical problem and it had stopped. This was huge! Talk about bringing a smile to my face. It was intriguing to see how the process of hypnosis paired with neuroplasticity could access areas of the brain to stop the continuous signals being sent out.

On Wednesday the pain or 'comfort level' in my back had dropped down to a zero for the first time since onset. I was excited but leery at the same time. It was a major move in the right direction.

Thursday morning I was scheduled for a massage. To be honest, I was a bit reluctant and worried walking to that appointment due to the fact that I had not been able to tolerate a massage on my back since 2011 when CRPS had moved into that area. I knew that my 'Comfort Level' had already dropped to a ZERO in my back, but I wasn't sure if I trusted it enough to do the massage. I was pleasantly surprised to see how relaxed and comfortable I was during the massage. I had no pain in my back and I was able to keep my 'Comfort Level' at a zero. To me this was a test, and it showed me what I had accomplished to that point was holding and would continue to get better.

As the week progressed we continued to hone in on the areas where I continued to have pain. Specifically my left foot and ankle. I was hoping and wishing for the best outcome – to walk away pain free – but I was afraid to get my hopes up. Little did I know, although I had hoped and prayed it would be, that my entire body would drop to a ZERO by the end of the week!

Yes, it was an intense week of learning, working, and following all of the instructions given me, but to have my pain drop to ZERO for the first time since 2006 when I sprained my ankle, then was diagnosed with CRPS, it was well worth it.

One of the things that I learned was that every cell has a memory. It is essential to provide the cells with a new memory other than pain, and when you do this, new memories will take hold as the cells regenerate every 90 days. Thus, in approximately 90 days after arriving home, new memories should be strong.

I was excited for the future. Finally!

CHAPTER 16

Lessons Learned

Throughout my journey with CRPS I learned so much. It was a journey filled with highs and lows, but I learned how important it was to set in place a new outlook on life too.

Positive Mindset

It is easy for chronic pain patients (myself included) to employ negative self-talk. *"My body is broken." "I feel like I'm 100 years old." "Life will never get better."* We say these things to ourselves multiple times a day when we are in pain and associate comments with our pain *"broken, old, and never getting better."*

What so many people don't realize is that during this process, the brain is creating a folder named, "Pain" that is filtering your words. In the folder is a stored document called *"Broken"*, another document called *"Old"*, and other called *"Never Get Better"*. The more we make negative comments about our pain, the more our brain keeps creating documents and saving them. The folder is becoming full of negative associations. When we have a pain flare, the folder pulls up the documents to help us interpret what we are feeling. Messages such as broken, old, and never getting better are retrieved and we feel worse. Then we say, "*It's no use. I will be living with this pain the rest of my life.*" Essentially, we are using our words to create a negative mindset towards our pain.

What is going on? The billions of neurons in the brain form connections with other neurons to send signals in the brain. As a group of neurons grows, so does the ability to send messages throughout the brain. In that process, the nervous system creates memories or what are called neurosignatures of neurotags. A neurotag is simply a pattern of neuron activation that creates outputs in the brain. Those outputs can be perception, thought, movement, or immune responses. [14] This is how the brain remembers what it learns.

You may have heard the saying "*Neurons that fire together, wire together.*" Neurons become activated (fire) and link together (wire) to interpret a signal input from a neurotag and can trigger memory. Neurotags form and strengthen through repetition and in other ways. Eventually, neurons can fire at just the thought of something.

Pain is an output of a physical linking of neurotags at a particular time. We are not conscious of this process, but we have a very personalized neurosignature for pain. [15] Thoughts and emotions are connected to neurotag networks and can become sensitized and remembered. For example, a neurotag for CRPS pain may be associated with one called "sprain". When the sprain neurotag is activated, it is likely that the CRPS pain neurotag will also be activated. Thus, thinking about a sprain can activate pain.

According to pain specialist G. Lorimer Moseley, we can create and modify our neurotags in many ways. [16] Moving in new ways to stimulate the nervous system is one example. We can also change our pain associations by being positive about pain and not creating negative associations. Yes, this is easier said then done.

We have a growth mindset, you can grow, overcome adversity, and change your pain. Pain doesn't have to define you. It's a problem to be faced. As you change your thoughts and behaviors, you change your brain. With a growth mindset, you can live beyond pain. Mindset matters when dealing with chronic pain and it makes a difference in how we feel. This is part of creating a positive neurosignature.

If you expect to feel worse, to not get better, to have life ruined by pain, you have a negative (fixed) mindset that will keep you stagnant and in pain. Such expectations prime your nervous system for more pain. They will also undermine your recovery and enhance your pain.

Instead you want to prime your brain for pain relief. For example, if you are thinking, 'I can't increase my activity because it will create a pain flare', you are priming your brain for more pain. However, if you think, 'I can slowly increase my activity and I will feel good', you are priming your brain for a pain relief. Positive expectations will push you forward to grow. They will start to override or erase the old documents in the folder and replace them with new documents.

If you refuse to give in to your pain and refuse to believe you will never get better and fight back with all the tools you are given, you will create a growth mindset. Maybe you haven't solved all the issues yet, but you are working on them one by one. Remember the importance of small positive steps forward. The goal is to thrive, not simply survive, so here are a few more ways to develop a positive mindset while dealing with chronic pain.

Use Positive Affirmations

It is important to remind yourself daily that you are not your pain. Don't allow pain to take over your life and dominate your thoughts. If you think only negative thoughts, you will see only negative. Here are a few positive affirmations to help you create a more positive approach to pain.

I am calm, I am comfortable, I am in control.

I learn from every situation.

I am strong, courageous and confident.

I can get through this.

I inhale confidence and exhale fear.

You are entirely up to YOU. Make your body. Make your health. Make your life. Make yourself.

I have the power to change myself. My body is an amazing healer.

Begin your day with a positive affirmation. Think about things in your life that are positive and good. This is an intentional process of focusing your mind on a positive aspect of your life when you start your day. By saying positive affirmations, you are training your brain to focus on things of joy, positive experiences, etc. Every day you can find positive things to focus on if you look. It won't make the pain disappear, but it will help your experience of pain.

Practice Gratitude

You might be thinking, *I am in pain. Why should I be grateful?* Because there are so many other parts of your life – moments and experiences – that are positive. Gratitude is a state of mind of thankfulness and appreciation. It is an attitude, something that most of us must cultivate because it is easy to focus on negatives. Practicing gratitude doesn't mean you ignore your pain. That is impossible. Rather, you choose not to let it define you or your day.

Think of it as planting positive seeds and pulling the weeds in our mind. Positive seeds are the equivalent to gratitude. Weeds are the negative thoughts that can pile up and only stop our seeds from growing. When we can pull the weeds from our garden in our mind, then our seeds can flourish!

When we express gratitude, it makes us feel good. It creates positive emotions and even feeling of happiness. One reason for this is that expressing gratitude can release the bonding hormone oxytocin. [17] This physiological release decreases the release of stress hormones, such as cortisol, and promotes health. The science of gratitude is linked to a hold of health benefits. Gratitude has been shown to lower blood pressure and boost the immune system related to cardiac health, to name just a few. [18]

Practicing gratitude has also been linked to better sleep. [19] Try being grateful and focus on the blessings of the day before you go to sleep. Doing so relaxes you and puts you in a positive frame of mind. The more you focus on the positives of your day, the less worry and negativity will fill your mind.

Gratitude can also decrease feelings of depression and anxiety. [20] Focusing on what you appreciate about others and about your life puts you in a positive state of mind and can help you fall asleep.

To better illustrate the effects of gratitude, consider a study conducted by researchers Robert Emmons and Michael McCullough, who wanted to see if gratitude would have an influence on well-being. They compared three groups of people:

1. Those in one group kept a gratitude journal.
2. Those in the second group focused on negative life events (or what they called hassles).
3. Those in the third group focused on neutral events.

What they discovered was that the people in the gratitude-focused group felt better about their lives, were more optimistic, and reported fewer physical complaints. In addition, the gratitude group had improvement in sleep in that they got more hours of sleep at night. [21]

You don't have to keep a gratitude journal, but some people find that a journal helps them focus. And the benefit of a journal is that on a bad pain day, you can go back and read an entry that will remind you of your blessings. You are not denying your pain but rather choosing to focus on the things in your day that are positive. The change in focus away from pain helps you feel better.

An easy way to begin practicing gratitude is to do so at the beginning and end of your day. Think of three things you can count as a blessing. At first, doing this might be difficult simply because you are not used to this focus. But over time, it will be easier because you will be more tuned in to finding the positives. In fact, a focus on gratitude can be learned.

To help you get started practicing gratitude, here are some ideas from people living with chronic pain who know the importance of gratitude in terms of keeping their outlook positive.

1. Start noticing any small thing that brings you pleasure or joy. Don't negate anything in the process. Something as inconsequential as light traffic on the way home can be noticed.
2. Start a gratitude challenge with a friend or family member. If you want to improve good feelings towards someone, this can help.
3. Use mindfulness and make a blessing the focus.
4. Journal your gratitude moments and read through them regularly to remind you of your many blessings.
5. Write a thank-you note to people, especially those who have contributed to your life. This could even be a quick

text message.

6. Set a goal to express gratitude to one or two people a day.

7. Make a gratitude jar and have anyone who lives with you contribute slips of paper in the jar. Periodically, pull out slips of paper and read them. This is an exercise often done at Thanksgiving, but it can be done all year.

8. Smile and disrupt the flow of negativity. Flashing a smile can be a visual reminder that there is much to be happy about in life, despite the challenges you are currently facing.

Learn to Forgive

When we live with pain, it is tempting to listen to the small voice whispering in your ear, "*Why you? This isn't fair. You don't deserve this. No one understands.*" The result of such thoughts can be resentment and even bitterness. Both can lead to self-pity and misery. A way to protect yourself is to make forgiveness a part of a positive mindset.

Most people living with chronic pain (myself included) can find this a challenge. But it is an important step in the healing process.

People who treat chronic pain report that some patients have trouble forgiving people whom they feel have offended them in some way. [22] And when unforgiveness is present, chronic pain goes up. Unforgiveness has an impact on the physical body via the nervous and endocrine systems. The distress associated with unforgiveness can be transformed into pain. But forgiveness can promote health. [23]

One of the reasons why people struggle with forgiveness is because they misunderstand it. They think it means accepting what the person did or convincing themselves that what happened was not hurtful. That is not the case. It is about making a conscious decision to break the chains from the past and to allow yourself to move forward. In other words, not allowing the people, events or things in the past to dictate your future. Forgiveness is an action within our control.

To develop a positive mindset - use positive affirmations, practice gratitude, and learn to forgive. Such actions involve areas of your life over which you can exercise control and can lead to positive emotions and attitudes that can help you live beyond pain and begin to regain your life.

All of these things can and will help you work with neuroplasticity too. Think of it this way – If you have a horse in a city, they put blinders on it to keep it from getting distracted by the pedestrians and cars. In much the same way our brain essentially puts blinders on us when we are dealing with chronic pain. We are so focused on the minute, the hours and getting through the day that a positive mindset, gratitude, forgiveness and positive moments are forgotten. When we start practicing these things and reminding ourselves of the positive it allows us to take off the blinders and reopen the doors that need to be opened.

CHAPTER 17

New Lease on Life

I was so sure of myself flying home that I cancelled the wheelchair assistance. I wanted to do this on my own. I had my cane if I needed it, but I was feeling pretty darn confident.

The plane ride home was full of excitement and trepidation at the same time. I was ecstatic to be sitting in an airplane pain free on my way home. On the other hand I had thoughts running through my head about how I could pick up the pieces to move forward. This was an adjustment. Not only did my body need time to adjust so did I from an emotional perspective.

When I arrived home I was barraged with questions, because friends and family members immediately noticed a marked difference in my demeanor, a bigger smile on my face, my ability to put weight on my left foot for the first time since 2006, and an overall sense of well-being. This was after 5 days' worth of treatment with hypnosis in a multi-therapeutic approach. Yes, there were some people that were skeptical and others that were true believers. The bottom line is – seeing is believing.

Once settled, I put myself into a routine that included listening to the CDs of the sessions that I had completed, doing self-hypnosis, and utilizing the tools given to me from my intensive. After the first week home, I was no longer utilizing my cane to walk. I still needed to work on my gait, but this was a big milestone.

During this time, I also met with my Dr. Amir. He was used to me going to Germany for treatment and coming back with their protocols, but this time he had no idea what to expect. When he entered the exam room, I was sitting there with socks and running shoes on, no cane and long pants that could touch my ankle and medial side of my foot.

My Pain Management doctor looked at me, pushed back on his stool, and started looking around the room. He was in disbelief at what he was seeing. He then asked me to take off my left shoe and sock, because he wanted to see if my left little toe was still spasming or doing the rhythmical movement. When he saw that it was not moving, my coloration was not off in my foot, and I was feeling great, he was dumbfounded. His next words were, "*I'm being punked. Where are the cameras and how are you doing this?*" I had to laugh. He wanted to know what I did in my treatments, but since he didn't fully understand what I did, he was skeptical. Then when I asked him to take me off of my pain medications, he was awestruck. He hesitated, to say the least, because he wasn't sure this was going to hold. As I told him, I am confident in where I am and what I have accomplished. I have no pain at this time, so I don't feel that I should continue on pain medications, and I asked again to be titrated off of them.

Week by week, I continued to see progress. Having the ability to walk my dog at the park with no pain, completely comfortable, completing household chores with no discomfort, babysitting my nephew who was 6 months old with complete confidence, and spending time with my family in activities that I would not have been able to have done previously. These are all the rewards of utilizing neuroplasticity training, learning self-hypnosis and following through with what I was taught during my treatment.

The weeks turned into months and I realized how precious life was. I had the opportunity to regain my life and that was a true blessing. It got me thinking about what I had missed out on and what I had to look forward to. At this point it was more about staying in the present and looking toward the future.

Every morning the sunrise seemed more meaningful. Watching a butterfly flutter through the air in a carefree way struck a chord. Turning the music up when no one was home, singing and dancing around the house – truly amazing! I was learning how to embrace life again, only with more meaning and zeal.

It was during this time that I contacted Ron and we talked about me taking the steps to get credentialed and certified as a Clinical Hypnotist. Ron trains a plethora of people but no one had ever replicated what he did. I felt there was a big enough need that this needed to be done, so I put the ball in motion.

A little over three months after getting into remission I signed up for my first 5k. I felt like I needed to prove to myself and to everyone around me that I was ok. There weren't any grandioso ideas that I would be able to run the whole thing. I just had a goal of doing a walk / jog and finishing it. That would be an accomplishment in itself, and I did it!

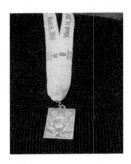

CHAPTER 18

Giving Back

Wow, I was high on life. It felt like all the pieces of my puzzle had come together and I was on a brand new path. A path of excitement, enlightenment, empowerment, and more than anything wanting to give back to the chronic pain community.

Five months after getting into complete remission from my CRPS (which I had been told *"would end my life as I knew it"*) I was completing my credentials and certifications as a Clinical Hypnotist. I was so excited! This was the first step towards helping other CPRS and chronic pain patients in much the same way that I was helped. I knew in my heart that there was a huge need and something more had to be offered to others so they didn't have to go through everything that I did.

Once back home from my training I starting putting the pieces in place to open up my office. I wanted to make sure that I had everything that I would need with regard to training, business, marketing and understanding. I jumped in with both feet to get additional credentials in Pain Management, Cancer Patient Care, PTSD and Palliative Care. I felt that these added with my experience as a CRPS patient would make a well-rounded package.

Since gaining remission in 2013 I have continued to be completely pain free and have had the ability to regain my life. It is important for people living with CRPS and other chronic pain conditions to hear about positive outcomes such as mine. This is not a one off or something that cannot happen to others. As a matter of fact, I am honored to say that I have treated hundreds of other CRPS and chronic pain patients many of whom have had the same outcome.

I have put together a protocol called - HCT (Hypnosis Combined Therapy). This protocol is very similar to what helped me get into remission with some exciting changes based upon medical advancements and new technology. HCT is a multi-modality protocol that is evidence based, non-invasive and drug free. Individualizing this protocol to meet the specific needs of each patient and treating them as a whole is key to them meeting their goals. For some, success is gaining functional levels where they can live their life. While others have gained full long-term remission are continuing to thrive.

Chronic pain is more than just the physical pain. It is also the emotional, mental, and spiritual aspects of life that need to be addressed too. Therefore an individualized protocol that address all aspects of what a chronic pain patient is going through is key to long-term success.

I've had the privilege of treating chronic pain patients (CRPS, AMPS, phantom limb pain, Fibromyalgia, neuropathic pain, chronic migraines, Lyme, neuropathy, back pain, etc.) from around the world. Each person comes with their own journey of living with chronic pain. Then they leave with their personal tale of transformation: regaining function, meeting goals, increasing their restorative sleep, and having the tools to move forward to live their life. This is amazing to say the least.

Yes, I have a different perspective on chronic pain, CRPS and pain control than most people you will meet. We may not have a cure for CRPS, but I ask people all the time, *"What is the difference between long-term remission, being able to live your life, and a cure?"* Right now, long-term remission is the most obvious choice until we have major advancements in research and science.

Personally, I believe that you have to stay ahead of the curve to make sure that the most innovative, scientific and evidence based treatments are available to chronic pain patients. This is exactly what I've done with HCT. I trained with and put in place, the same protocols that got me into long-term remission and then added in additional modalities based upon the latest scientific advances, technology, and outcomes. It is this combination that is giving patients outstanding outcomes with a protocol that doesn't come with a list of negative side-effects.

I know for some it is hard to believe, but trust me - with everything that I went through with treatments in the United States (Traditional Western Medicine), in Frankfurt, German (Integrative Medicine), Mexico (Integrative Medicine), and then back to the US to be treated with Mind-Body medicine for pain management - I think I can say I looked at everything, tried just about everything. I eventually found what worked for me. I have heard from others with CRPS that they have tried hypnosis and it just doesn't work. I too tried hypnosis prior to going back to be treated in 2013, my previous treatments with hypnosis didn't help me either – then again they were not well versed in chronic pain and not certified in 'Pain Management' either. The right combination was finding someone well versed in chronic pain, pain management and clinical hypnosis.

HCT is a completely different way of looking at things, working with chronic pain, individualizing a protocol, treating the person as a whole, and finding a solution for the pain. What works for one will not necessarily work for all, but if it is successful for one it is likely going to be successful for many. It is important for each chronic pain patient to find a treatment protocol that they are comfortable with and they feel will help them to regain their life. Information can be the most valuable tool we have in helping us make a huge difference in the lives of those living with chronic pain and CRPS.

CHAPTER 19

Caregivers and Patients

Caregivers

Being a caregiver is one of the most difficult and demanding jobs. It is a matter of balancing the needs of the patient or a loved one while providing him or her with a path to the outside world. CRPS and chronic pain are conditions that can cause isolation, frustration, stress, anxiety, depression and/or PTSD. That is a lot for anyone to cope with.

Knowing how to address your loved one's needs can take some time and patience. This also involves setting healthy boundaries so that you can make sure to keep yourself whole and healthy too. Knowledge is power. The more you know - about the diagnosis, current treatments, potential treatments, side effects of medications - the more empowered you are. Remember, you have to take care of yourself in order to take care of others.

Understanding a diagnosis and how it can affect

each person can make life much easier. What is a pain cycle? How can he or she be capable for several hours, and be hit with debilitating pain for the rest of the day?

Chronic pain, more specifically CRPS, tends to fluctuate in intensity. There will be many weeks where it seems like you've taken two steps forward and one step back. Knowing that your loved one's well-being can constantly shift from high to low. The key is understanding this process is normal, reducing the shift or fluctuation to ensure a steadier flow, and perceiving just how sensitive the patient is to their surrounding or circumstances will help.

Utilizing pain-intensity scales or better yet, 'comfort scales' will help you gain a better understanding of the type and degree of pain that he or she is experiencing on a given day or a given time. The McGill Pain Index from McGill University has been used to help gauge the intensity of CRPS pain and other conditions. (Figure 1) Created in 1971, this index illustrates types and levels of pain for various conditions, presenting a coherent consistency in various aspects of pain that doctors use around the world. Note, you will see 'causalgia' which is Complex Regional Pain Syndrome (Type 2); this is Latin for burning pain; found in both CRPS type 1 (RSD) and CRPS type 2 (causalgia).

** Figure 1

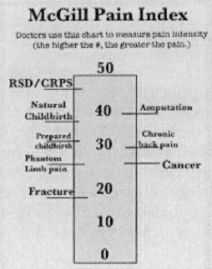

McGill Pain Index

Doctors use this chart to measure pain intensity
(the higher the #, the greater the pain.)

50

RSD/CRPS

Natural Childbirth — 40 — Amputation

Prepared childbirth — 30 — Chronic back pain

Phantom Limb pain — — Cancer

Fracture — 20

10

0

Triggers and Stressors

Stress, anxiety, fear, frustration, isolation and anticipation are all a common thread in CRPS and chronic pain patients. The more the patient can have a sense of calm, security and control – the better off they will be. Knowing what the triggers are that cause the stress, anxiety, fear, and anticipation can help you to put things in place to diminish or control a reaction. Stress and anxiety have been proven to increase pain and they can have other negative side effects on the patient's health. This is something to remember for yourself as well.

Find new ways to distract or calm down the patient or loved one, to keep them on track. Meditation, abdominal breathing, self-hypnosis or even music can be useful tools and outlets for both the patient and caregiver.

Weather and Climate

Weather is a common complaint that affects pain levels. Climate changes, changes in the season, weather patterns – these all impact the barometric pressure and often cause an increase in discomfort. Sometimes it is just a subtle shift, but other times it can cause a complete flare. You can use the weather to guide your dialogue in regards to the patient's needs and pain level.

Other Considerations

Many times something as small as a draft from the air conditioner, a bump in a car or the vibration can cause pain to reverberate through your loved one's body. Help decrease an anticipatory stress or anxiety by being aware of these items and being proactive. Be aware of the things that can cause an increase in discomfort and suggest alternatives to help the individual feel more at ease.

Certain foods, drinks or chemicals such as caffeine, alcohol and nitrates can causes added irritation. Knowing what affects a person or how they react can help diminish any flare and keep things on an even keel.

Relationships are a lifeline for a chronic pain patient. Therefore, a lack of balance in relationships becomes all the more distressing. Try to let petty issues go and find a healthy way to communicate. Open communication is always key to any healthy relationship.

If you ever feel that you have too much on your plate as a caregiver – there is a way to make assistance really matter. If you need a break then make the time to take care of you. Remember, your feelings are just as valid.

It's important to understand that the person with chronic pain or CRPS also needs to learn how to plan, verbalize and move forward with simple tasks that he or she could do without thinking. Knowing how to utilize time and move forward productively take time for both the caregiver and patient. In fact, it requires a new pattern of thought in the patient's case.

Independence and Dips in the Road

As your loved one begins to regain their independence and starts to take back responsibilities, their journey will continue to require your support. There can be times when this support may come in different ways. Many times chronic pain patients will experience anger, frustration, sadness and resentment that can cloud their recovery due to the adaptations necessary to accomplish something that was easily done prior to their diagnosis. The thoughts and frustration of additional effort needed to complete a task, not being able to complete a project like before – these are common exasperations. When people are healing their emotions can be just as volatile as during the onset of their diagnosis, due to changes taking place and challenging frustration in their journey to regaining their life.

A Walk in Their Shoes

Being a caregiver, partner or spouse to someone diagnosed with chronic pain or CRPS can be daunting. It requires clear communication about changes taking place and what the future holds. Having the ability to be aware of the challenges, experiences and frustrations on all sides (caregiver, partner, spouse and/or patient) are important in sustaining a healthy relationship.

We all know it is not possible to walk a mile in someone else's shoes, but we can take a step back and look at what they are going through. What are their concerns, fears, frustrations, and struggles? What would it be like to have to deal with those 24/7? This is a two way street. Both individuals (patient and caregiver) need to be willing to walk in the shoes of the other. To see what it is like. To think about what the other person is experiencing. Then and only then can you come together as a stronger unit.

Understanding and Taking Care of Yourself

When you fly one of the first things the flight attendant goes over is if there is an emergency and the oxygen masks drop, secure your mask before trying to help anyone else. This is very true as a caregiver. You must take care of yourself in order to take care of others.

Adapting to a caretaker roll for someone with chronic pain or CRPS is difficult, regardless of the severity of the condition. As much as your loved one needs you, remember that being the best person you can be for him or her must include taking steps to keep yourself whole and healthy.

No matter how strong you are, how vigilant you are, how much effort you put in, or how tough you think you are the negative emotions hitting your loved one will also find their way to you. This is normal. But don't let anger, grief, guilt or fears hold you back. It's important to know that these feelings are a normal part of the process.

Take the time to nurture yourself. Whether it is

a support group, going to the gym, yoga, meditation, taking a spa day, or just a few hours to regenerate each night. Find the thing that will work for you to help you in the long run.

TREATMENT OPTIONS

(Referenced in alphabetical order.)

Acupuncture:
Acupuncture is one of the main forms of treatment in traditional Chinese medicine. It involves the use of sharp, thin needles that are inserted in the body at very specific points. This process is believed to adjust and alter the body's energy flow into healthier patterns and is used to treat a wide variety of illnesses and health conditions.
https://www.acupuncturetoday.com/mpacms/at/article.php?id=27704

Biofeedback:
Biofeedback is a technique you can use to learn to control some of your body's functions, such as your heart rate. During biofeedback, you're connected to a sensor(s) that help you receive information about your body. This feedback helps you make subtle changes in your body, such as relaxing certain muscles, to achieve the results you want, such as reducing pain. In essence, biofeedback gives you the ability to practice new ways to control your body, often to improve a health condition.
https://www.mayoclinic.org/tests-procedures/

biofeedback/about/pac-20384664

Blocks:

Lumbar Sympathetic Block:

A lumbar sympathetic block is an injection of medication that helps relieve lower back or leg pain. It can be used to treat: Reflex sympathetic dystrophy; Complex regional pain syndrome; Herpes zoster infection (shingles) involving the legs; Vascular insufficiency; Peripheral neuropathy

Stellate Ganglion Block:

The stellate ganglion is part of the sympathetic nervous system that is located in your neck, on either side of your voice box. A stellate ganglion block is an injection of medication into these nerves that can help relieve pain in the head, neck, upper arm and upper chest. It also can help increase circulation and blood supply to the arm.

Calmare aka Scrambler Therapy:

Calmare Therapy® (scrambler therapy) is a non-invasive, drug-free treatment for pain control and medication-resistant neuropathy. It uses biophysical "scrambler" technology, a treatment for nerve pain that uses electrodes placed on the skin. The device works to relieve pain directly at the pain site without any reliance on medication.

http://scramblertherapy.org/clinical-trials.htm

http://www.mattioli1885journals.com/

index.php/actabiomedica/article/
view/4306/3288

Cold Laser:
Cold laser therapy is low-intensity laser therapy that stimulates healing while using low levels of light.
The technique is called "cold" laser therapy because the low levels of light aren't enough to heat your body's tissue. The level of light is low when compared to other forms of laser therapy. Medical professionals use cold laser therapy in a variety of ways. The main uses for cold laser therapy are tissue repair and relief from pain and inflammation.

https://www.painnewsnetwork.org/
stories/2015/11/23/low-level-laser-therapy-for-
chronic-pain

EMDR:
Eye Movement Desensitization and Reprocessing (EMDR) therapy is an interactive psychotherapy technique used to relieve psychological stress. It is an effective treatment for chronic pain, trauma and post-traumatic stress disorder (PTSD).

https://www.healthline.com/health/emdr-
therapy

HCT Intensive:

HCT is a multi-modality, evidence based, non-invasive and drug free protocol that is individualized to meet each patient's specific needs (physically, mentally, emotionally, and spiritually). This is a combination of clinical hypnosis / medical hypnosis, biofeedback, cold laser, PEMF, light/sound therapy, neuroplasticity training, working with the limbic system, cell memory, and more. HCT has given patients, on an international basis, the ability to dramatically decrease pain levels (many gain long-term remission), increase restorative sleep, decrease and control stress, anxiety and/or PTSD, and regain their lives.

HCT is an Intesive that can range from 1 to 2 weeks (based upon the needs of the patient and location of Intensive), and is followed by a 90-day home program. HCT has an 85% success rate.

https://www.omicsonline.org/proceedings/the-effectiveness-of-using-hypnosis-combined-therapy-hct-for-the-treatment-of-chronic-pain-crps-fibromyalgia-neuropathic-50361.html

http://www.AdvancedPathways.com

Hypnosis:

Hypnosis is a mental state of highly focused concentration, diminished peripheral awareness, and heightened suggestibility. There are numerous techniques that experts employ for inducing such a state. Capitalizing on the power of suggestion, hypnosis is often used to help people relax, to diminish the sensation of pain, or to facilitate some desired behavioral change.

Therapists bring about hypnosis (also referred to as hypnotherapy or hypnotic suggestion) with the help of mental imagery and soothing verbal repetition that ease the patient into a trancelike state. Once relaxed, patients' minds are more open to transformative messages.

http://www.apa.org/research/action/
hypnosis.aspx

Hyperbaric Oxygen Therapy (HBOT):
Hyperbaric oxygen therapy (HBOT) is a medical treatment which enhances the body's natural healing process by inhalation of 100% oxygen in a total body chamber, where atmospheric pressure is increased and controlled. It is used for a wide variety of treatments usually as a part of an overall medical care plan.

http://rsds.org/wp-content/uploads/2015/02/
hbot_jintlmedresearch.pdf

Ketamine:
The anesthetic ketamine is used to treat various chronic pain syndromes, especially those that have a neuropathic component. Low dose ket-

amine produces strong analgesia in neuropathic pain states, presumably by inhibition of the N-methyl-D-aspartate receptor although other mechanisms are possibly involved, including enhancement of descending inhibition and anti-inflammatory effects at central sites.

https://www.ncbi.nlm.nih.gov/pubmed/23432384

http://rsdfoundation.org/en/Ketamine_Treatment.html

Neridronate:
Neridronate, or neridronic acid, is an amino-bisphosphonate (BP) used in Italy and most recently in the US to treat several bone diseases, e.g. Paget's disease of bone, osteogenesis imperfecta (OI), and complex regional pain syndrome (CRPS). Neridronate can be administrated intravenously, which means it is a valid option for those who cannot receive BPs orally.

https://www.ncbi.nlm.nih.gov/pmc/articles/PMC4632140/

http://www.vitality101.com/health-a-z/CRPS-new-highly-effective-treatment-for-crps

Neurofeedback:
Neurofeedback (NFB), also called neurotherapy or neurobiofeedback, is a type of biofeedback that uses real-time displays of brain activity—most commonly electroencephalography (EEG)—in an attempt to teach self-regulation of brain function.

https://www.researchgate.net/publication/233203234_Neurofeedback_Treatment_for_Pain_Associated_with_Complex_Regional_Pain_Syndrome_Type_I

Neuroplasticity Training:
Neuroplasticity, also known as brain plasticity, or neural plasticity, is the ability of the brain to change continuously throughout an individual's life, e.g., brain activity associated with a given function can be transferred to a different location, the proportion of grey matter can change and synapses may strengthen or weaken over time. The aim of neuroplasticity is to optimize the neural networks during phylogenesis, ontogeny and physiological learning, as well as after a brain injury. Research in the latter half of the 20th century showed that many aspects of the brain can be altered (or are "plastic") even through adulthood. However, the developing brain exhibits a higher degree of plasticity than the adult brain.

https://www.ncbi.nlm.nih.gov/pmc/articles/

PMC4922795/

http://rsds.org/wp-content/
uploads/2015/05/2015-brain-neuroplastic-
changes.pdf

Occupational Therapy:
Occupational therapy (OT) is the use of assess-
ment and intervention to develop, recover, or
maintain the meaningful activities, or occupa-
tions, of individuals, groups, or communities. It
is an allied health profession performed by occupational therapists and occupational therapy as-
sistants (OTA). OTs often work with people with
mental health problems, disabilities, injuries, or
impairments.

https://www.aota.org/about-occupational-
therapy/professionals/hw/articles/chronic-
pain.aspx

Physical Therapy:
Physical therapy (PT), also known as physiother-
apy, is one of the allied health professions that,
by using evidence-based kinesiology, electrother-
apy, shockwave modality, exercise prescription,
joint mobilization and health education, treats
conditions such as chronic or acute pain, soft
tissue injuries, cartilage damage, arthritis, gait

disorders and physical impairments typically of musculoskeletal, cardiopulmonary, neurological and endocrinological origins.

http://rsdguide.com/physical-therapy/

Spinal Cord Stimulator and DRG (Dorsal Root Ganglion) Stimulator:
A Spinal Cord Stimulator (SCS) or Dorsal Column Stimulator (DCS) is a type of implantable neuro-modulation device (sometimes called a "pain pacemaker") that is used to send electrical signals to select areas of the spinal cord (dorsal columns) for the treatment of certain pain conditions. SCS is a consideration for people who have a pain condition that has not responded to more conservative therapy.

https://academic.oup.com/bja/
article/92/3/348/310917/Spinal-cord-stimulation-in-complex-regional-pain

http://www.medgadget.com/2016/02/st-jude-medicals-axium-drg-stimulator-approved-by-fda-for-complex-regional-pain-syndrome.html

https://www.ncbi.nlm.nih.gov/
pubmed/21371254

Vecttor:
VECTTOR treatments are a form of electro-stimulation based upon acupuncture, physiology, cel-

lular physiology, and anatomy designed to stimulate the nerves to produce certain neuropeptides essential for optimal functioning of the body. These neuropeptides are vital for increasing circulation to the skin, bones nerves, muscles, and for reducing oxidative stress. The VECTTOR system is designed to read feedback from the body via skin surface temperatures, throughout the treatment process.

http://www.vecttor.com/

NOTES

(references and abbreviations)

References:

1. Institute of Medicine, Relieving, Pain in America: A Blueprint for Transforming Prevention, Care, Education, and Research (Washington, DC: National Academics Press, 2011), https://www.nap.edu/read/13172/chapter/2.
2. "AAPM Facts and Figures on Pain," American Academy of Pain Medicine, 2017, https://biomotionlabs.com/wp-content/uploads/2011/09/AAPM-Facts-Figures-on-Pain.pdf
3. "Global Pain Management Market of Reach US$60 Billion by 2015, According to a New Report by Global Industry Analysts, Inc.," PRWeb, https://www.prweb.com/releases/2011/prweb8052240.htm
4. "Overview of Chronic Pain Treatment," American Chronic Pain Association, 2018, https://www.theacpa.org/wp-content/uploads/2018/03/ACPA_Resource_Guide_2018-Final-v2.pdf
5. John J. Bonica, "Important Clinical Aspects of Acute and Chronic Pain," in Mechanisms of Pain and Analgesic Compounds, eds. Roland F. Beers and Edward Graham Bassett (New York: Raven Press, 1979), 15-29.

6. K.P. Grichnik and F. M. Ferrante, "The Difference between Acute and Chronic Pain," Mount Sinai Journal of Medicine 58, no. 3 (May 1991); 217-20.

7. John J. Bonica, et al., The Management of Pain (Philadelphia: Lea and Febiger, 1990)

8. Katarina Dedovic, et al., "The Brain and the Stress Axis: The Neural Correlates of Cortisol Regulation in Response to Stress," NeuroImage 47, no. 3 (2009): 864-71, doi: 10.1016/j.neuroimage.2009.05.074

9. M.N. Baliki et al., "Chronic Pain and the Emotional Brain: Specific Brain Activity Associated with Spontaneous Fluctuations of Intensity of Chronic Back Pain," Journal of Neuroscience 26, no. 47 (2006), doi: 10.1523/jneurosci.3576-06.2006.

10. Yang S, Chang MC. Chronic Pain: Structural and Functional Changes in Brain Structures and Associated Negative Affective States. Int J Mol Sci. 2019;20(13):3130. Published 2019 Jun 26. doi:10.3390/ijms20133130

11. Bruce S. McEwen, "Physiology and Neurobiology of Stress and Adaptation: Central Rose of the Brain, "Physiology Reviews 87, no. 3 (2007): 873-904, doi:10.1152/physrev.00041.2006.

12. Masafumi Morimoto et al., "Distribution of Glucocorticoid Receptor Immunoreactivity and MRNA in the Rat Brain: An Immunohistochemical and in Situ Hybridization Study," Neuroscience Research 26, no. 3 (1996): 235-69, doi:10.1016/s0168-0102(96)01105-4.

13. Etienne Vachon-Presseau et al., "The Stress

Model of Chronic Pain: Evidence from Basal Cortisol and Hippocampal Structure and Function in Humans," Brain 136, no. 3 (2013): 815-27, doi:10.1093/brain/aws371.

14. G. Lorimer Moseley and Johan W. S. Vlaeyen, "Beyond Nociception," Pain 156, no. 1(January 2015): 35-38, doi:10.1016/j.pain.00000000000000014.

15. David S. Butler and G. Lorimer Moseley, Explain Pain, 2nd ed. (Adelaide, Australia: Noigroup, 2013), 78.

16. Moseley and Vlaeyen, "Beyon Nociception."

17. Sara B. Algoe and Baldwin M. Way, "Evidence for a Role of the Oxytocin System, Indexed by Genetic Variation In CD38, in the Social Bonding Effects of Expressed Gratitude," Social Cognitive and Affective Neuroscience 9, no. 12 (January 2014): 1855-61, doi:10.1093/scan/nst182.

18. Paul J. Mills et al., "The Role of Gratitude in Spiritual Well-Being in Asymptomatic Heart Failure Patients," Spirituality in Clinical Practice 2, no. 1 (March 2015): 5-17, doi:10.1037/scp0000050.

19. Alex M. Wood et al., "Gratitude Influences Sleep through the Mechanism of Pre-Sleep Cognition," Journal of Psychosomatic Research 66, no. 1 (January 2009): 43-48, doi:10.1016/j.j-psychores.2008.09.002.

20. Mei Yee Ng and Wing Sze Wong, "The Differential Effects of Gratitude and Sleep on Psychological Distress in Patients with

Chronic Pain," Journal of Health Psychology 18, no. 2 (March 2012): 263-71, doi:10.1177/1359105312439733.

21. Robert A. Emmons and Michael E. McCullough, "Counting Blessings verses Burdens: An Experimental Investigation of Gratitude and Subjective Well-Being in Daily Life," Journal of Personality & Social Psychology 84, no. 2(2003): 377-89, doi:10.1037//0022-3514.84.2.377.

22. James W. Carson et al., "Forgiveness and Chronic Low Back Pain: A Preliminary Study Examining the Relationship of Forgiveness to Pain, Anger, and Psychological Distress," Journal of Pain 6, no. 2 (March 2005): 84-91, doi:10.1016/j-jpain.2004.10.1012.

23. Everett L. Worthington, Forgiveness and Reconciliation: Theory and Application (London: Routledge, 2006).

Abbreviations:

ACC	Anterior Cingulate Cortex
AMPS	Amplified Musculoskeletal Pain Syndrome
CAM	Controlled Ankle Movement
CRPS	Complex Regional Pain Syndrome
CT	Computerized Tomography
DME	Durable Medical Equipment
ER	Emergency Room
FDA	Food and Drug Administration
HBOT	Hyperbaric Oxygen Therapy

HCT	Hypnosis Combined Therapy
HPA	Hypothalamic Pituitary Adrenal
ICU	Intensive Care Unit
IPT	Insulin Potentiation Therapy
JAMA	Journal of the American Medical Association
LSB	Lumbar Sympathetic Block
MRI	Magnetic Resonance Imaging
NAc	Nucleus Accumbens
NSAIDS	Nonsteroidal anti-inflammatory
NWB	Non-Weight Bearing
OP	Operative (report)
OT	Occupational Therapy
PACU	Post Anesthesia Care Unit
PEMF	Pulsed Electromagnetic Field
PT	Physical Therapy
PTT	Posterior Tibial Tendon
RNA	Ribonucleic Acid
RSD	Reflex Sympathetic Dystrophy
SCS	Spinal Cord Stimulator
TENS	Transcutaneous Electrical Neuromuscular Stimulation
TTR	Tarsal Tunnel Release
VTA	Ventral Tegmental Area

Printed in Great Britain
by Amazon